ADVANCE PRAISE FOR *BAD MEDICINE*

"*Bad Medicine* is a must-read for anyone concerned about the future of America's healthcare system. In gripping detail, Steve Soloway illustrates the frightening realities we face and what the nation must do going forward to ensure our survival. He also shares the secrets patients need to know to live healthier and happier lives. Fascinating and enormously valuable, each chapter of this profound examination will be cited for years to come."

—Chris Christie, former New Jersey Governor

"*Bad Medicine* gives a comprehensive and in-depth look at the challenges the healthcare industry faces and best practices on how to navigate these challenges. A must-read for anyone looking for solutions to problems. I have a full understanding of issues, both political and non-political, that interfere with the healthcare delivery that we have. I, like others, assumed all doctors were the same. It's clearly elucidated through the brilliant writing of Doctor Soloway that this can't be further from the truth."

—Michael L. Testa, Jr., New Jersey State Senator

"A dose of raw in-your-face truth for anyone who can handle it. I've witnessed and experienced firsthand the atrocities described in this book. Due to negligent physicians, I was left with an outwardly visible tumor for two years before I was finally diagnosed with cancer. This book explains exactly how and why stories like mine are sadly more prevalent than not. It can help patients understand the ways the system is broken—giving them a chance to navigate it better!"

—Fame Cohen, owner, Fame Luxury Stone

"With his laser sharp intellect, instinct, and acute knowledge of medicine, business, and politics, Dr. Soloway brings a unique combination of power to the table. His words are sincere, succinct, and powerful. He speaks echoes of all the problems in today's world that need to be addressed. It offers great solutions. It was a great read."

—Rik Mehta, US Senate candidate

"A must-read! It is somewhat cathartic to have a medical professional shed light on what so many patients are experiencing and can't make sense of! Very informative and empowering!"

—**Sandy Cohen, New York/Hamptons artist**

"It truly is all about his patients and comfort of others. In the world of Bad Medicine many of you will realize that one good doctor, namely "Dr. Soloway" can make a difference in your own space and time and there is no room for anything but the best. The book is a fast enjoyable read!!"

—**Cindy Montgomery, renowned national designer**

"Eye opening and very sobering. Dr. Soloway has given the patient/consumer great insight into the world of medicine: past/present, and future. First-class work."

—**N. L. DePace, MD, FACC**

"Dr. Soloway is a true expert with chutzpah. You have to possess serious chutzpah to take on the medical industry—as you will see in his book. Stephen Soloway is 'New York brash' and his book provides vital insights into a subject where many lives are on the line, while remaining entertaining at the same time."

—**Michael W. Cutler, senior special agent, INS (Ret.)**

"This is the first and only book to reveal the perils of medicine today, and he reveals the shocking Truth. A MUST-READ."

—**Martha Boneta, President of Vote America First**

"Never have I read a book so truthfully sad yet informative to the medical underground! You will enjoy his blunt, direct, no-nonsense approach to medicine and the faults of our medical system as he sees it from an insider's view. I strongly recommend this book for anyone who wants to learn more about our medical system, arthritis, self-determination, and Never Giving Up."

—**George A. Dendrinos, MD**

"This book will be a catalyst for positive change as it will save lives and improve the quality of lives."

—**Christopher J. Lotz, self-employed**

BAD MEDICINE
THE HORRORS OF AMERICAN HEALTHCARE

BY DR. STEPHEN SOLOWAY

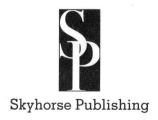

Skyhorse Publishing

Skyhorse Publishing books may be purchased in bulk at special discounts for sales promotion, corporate gifts, fund-raising, or educational purposes. Special editions can also be created to specifications. For details, contact the Special Sales Department, Skyhorse Publishing, 307 West 36th Street, 11th Floor, New York, NY 10018 or info@skyhorsepublishing.com.

Skyhorse® and Skyhorse Publishing® are registered trademarks of Skyhorse Publishing, Inc.®, a Delaware corporation.

Visit our website at www.skyhorsepublishing.com.

10 9 8 7 6 5 4 3 2 1

Library of Congress Cataloging-in-Publication Data is available on file.

Cover design by Mary Mohr, BuzzFactory
Cover photo credit: Stephen Soloway

ISBN: 978-1-5107-6243-5
Ebook ISBN: 978-1-5107-6245-9

Printed in the United States of America

CONTENTS

INTRODUCTION

My name is Dr. Stephen Soloway, and I'm the best.

The sharpshooter. The caviar. The Rolls Royce of Rheumatology.

Muhammad Ali called himself the greatest, and didn't win every fight, nor do I get a diagnosis 100 percent of the time! I'm totally one of a kind: a novel thinker, nonconformist, and after you read this book, I know you'll believe me.

Let's get one thing straight before we move forward: *Political correctness is killing our country.* Of course, that's not our only problem. (If it were, I wouldn't need three hundred pages to talk about it!) Political correctness is one of many societal trends that are crippling our great nation. We'll never solve them if people can't get serious. Let's get serious from the start: our country is in a tailspin, and our forefathers are rolling over in their graves.

I've never had a problem telling it like it is. Call it no filter, call me Archie Bunker, or call me Dr. Trump (as my Republican patients do). My mouth has always been my biggest ally and my biggest enemy.

I'm no bloviator, nor am I ultracrepidarian. I don't prevaricate, and I am supercilious. (Can you tell I am a lexicon?) In many cases, what I say could save your life.

I must share with you a story of my daily life. Patients come from near and far with serious health problems. It is rare that I get "easy" patients who have simple shoulder, knee, or back pain—or other easy problems, such as carpal tunnel syndrome, heel spurs, tennis elbow, trigger fingers, or plantar fasciitis, rotator cuff issues, and other things that we refer to as soft tissue rheumatism. Sadly, nobody can do the joints like me. I'm not practicing. I'm solving problems.

I intimidate patients due to my strong personality. (I'm actually a teddy bear.) I am humbled and sympathetic toward the needs of the patients. I emphasize to patients, "You have come to me with a problem. My plan or medication is a problem, as well. One problem is exchanged for another—untreated illness is worse than the potential side effects of a proposed treatment." I am very forthright with my patients, some of whom travel over three hours, or three days, to get here, then sit in the waiting room for another three hours. I understand this to be frustrating. They instilled trust in me by coming; however, sometimes they do not want to follow the plan. I ask that they keep this trust in me since they sought my expertise, and I explain that new medications have destroyed crippling arthritis. What I'm trying to tell you is that the crippling arthritis is so well treatable that it's better to have than the so-called good arthritis, which has fewer treatment options. It's unfortunate that some come only to vent and not to get better. Eventually, they come around and comprehend the plan, apologize, and wish they had started treatment sooner. This philosophy has now been working for thirty years.

Some don't appreciate the way I speak. Please understand that I am a New Yorker after all! Ah, but I saved your life! Well, yeah. So, did you come to me to make friends with you or to save your life? Which one is it?

Reading this book could save your life, and that's not an exaggeration. For the first time, I'm ready to tell the world the dirty truth about our country's medical system. More important, I'll tell you what you need to know to survive it, and how we can begin to fix it, too.

Nobody knows this better than I. Along my journey to the top—in no particular order—I have seen abuse, malpractice, malfeasance, fraud, waste, abuse, discrimination, good people, bad people, mistakes (many avoidable), scams, con artists, political hack jobs, and worse. Frankly, for the most part it all boils down to baloney.

Everyone believes that we have the best medical system in the world, because we have the most money. The lion's share of people don't understand the system, though, and the majority of the people running the system prefer it that way. They'll lie to your face if it means protecting their pockets.

Nobody tells the truth. Look at all these politicians. Everybody lies. They lie more than they break the speed limit, and everyone knows it, too. We're all in on the joke, but ultimately, the joke's on us.

Since the COVID-19 pandemic hit our country, however, nobody's laughing. It's clear that we need to get serious about what's going on in our hospitals, schools, and malls or countless will die. My one million predicted is at 300,000 and rising 1,000 per day.

I will tell you the truth about what really goes down in our medical system, from the top all the way to the bottom. Get ready—it will definitely make you sick.

CHAPTER 1
THE MAN, THE MYTH, THE LEGEND

At this point, you might be wondering: "Why should I listen to you?" I've treated many professional athletes, dignitaries, and celebrities, such as Lou "The Hulk" Ferrigno, who posted the visit on his Facebook. President Trump appointed me to the President's Council on Sports, Fitness & Nutrition. I've been appointed to the New Jersey Board of Medical Examiners by Governor Chris Christie. I've been named one of America's Top Doctors by *U.S. News & World Report*, and Castle Connolly, probably more times than anyone. I am the division chief of Rheumatology at the Inspira Health Network and designed the curriculum for my field at the institution, and I hold nine patents for devices in my field! I know the ins and outs of the healthcare system in our country from the bottom to the top. The system has been good to me. That in itself is a story worth repeating.

I grew up in Corona, Queens—where I was the minority. I had to walk vigilant and carefully through the streets to get to school—dreading every day the interval from Junction Boulevard to 99th Street, along 57th Avenue. When I dreamed big, I thought, "if I could only get a Corvette" I'd be the happiest person alive.

My mom was a housewife, and she and my dad gave me the best life I could have had. My dad took me ice skating in Central Park every Sunday and to Little League on Fleet Street. Mom took me to buy baseball cards every Friday—I loved baseball so much. I had always been a Mets fan. (At that age they thought I'd go pro, but my eyesight wasn't quite with the program.)

We were the typical middle-class family, and we had fun mixed with life lessons. We never had a pet, mom hated pets! (I had a fish, though.) I remember sledding off of the Long Island Expressway. It was the only hill we had.

We walked up this fifty- or seventy-foot hill, got to the top, realized we were a few feet from the right lane of traffic, heading toward Manhattan from Long Island on the crowded Long Island Expressway. Oblivious to the cars speeding by, I would jump on my sled and go down that hill and glide as long as I could before turning around to walk back up the hill yet again.

Saturdays, we'd go to see my mom's parents in Kew Gardens, or we'd visit my dad's parents in Flatbush. My dad's parents had both been born in the 1800s; to me, they were ancient. They started out raising chickens, but when that didn't go so well, my grandfather became an accountant. My dad's father had only one tooth (one-tooth John, or "dappy"). He kept the rest of his teeth in his pocket, and he'd always sneak me dark chocolate from the refrigerator. (I didn't stop to think the chocolate might be the cause of my grandfather's dental issues!) Meanwhile, my grandmother was wheelchair-bound. She had had a stroke at a young age and lived the rest of her life in a wheelchair. She'd give me a dollar every time I saw her, but they weren't made of money. They had another family living with them in their apartment: my dad's eldest sister, her husband, and two sons.

It was a happy childhood, but the road to medicine was desire and hard work—instilled in my mind from childhood. I was going to achieve more than my parents. I was going to be a doctor. I thought all the Jewish kids would be doctors. Many became doctors because they had to. Some (me) actually enjoyed it when we got there, though, and I for one loved it. It would take a while to get there.

I've been working in some fashion since I was thirteen. I couldn't count all my jobs. My first job was at Woolworths (stock boy). I was too young for working papers, so I was paid in cash: sometimes $6.00 a week, sometimes $20.00 a week. It depended on how much free time I had after school.

After that job, I made my way through the local economy. In no particular order: I was a lifeguard at a pool, and a caddy at a golf course; I picked up deliveries for specialty food stores; I scooped ice cream at an ice cream market; I was a camp counselor; I worked in a medical warehouse packing boxes and taking phone calls; I was a waiter at a catering hall; I did food prep at Benihana.

Later, I did paramedical exams. I drove all over Long Island—the entire LIE (Long Island Expressway), five hundred miles a day, making about twenty-five stops at about $10.00 a stop to draw blood, and I thought I was wealthy. I was feeling like Andy Warhol, in love with money.

I envied Warhol and Basquiat. They were colorful and so prolific. Warhol eventually had machines do the work, using ink instead of paint (genius). Today, I have a Warhol. Over time, I realized that I could have more success working for myself than working for somebody else. (My parents instilled this in me.)

My first true entrepreneurial venture came at a pretty young age, when I began selling ice cream at Jones Beach in high school. Sadly, my transportation was made possible because my grandfather's Parkinson's disease took his car, which became my car. I would buy dry ice, ice cream, and soda, carry it on the beach, and sell it all. Never a day passed that I didn't sell out. That was the summer operation. In the winter, I was shoveling snow sunup to sundown. The money that I made shoveling snow back in the seventies was the first money I started investing. I worked at a durable medical equipment company for two summers. Uncle Martin was a fair boss—he owned the place. In addition to getting close to my uncle, minimum wage was only two dollars per hour, and he paid more. (I went to Texas for that job!) At an early age, I had that ambition gene, that drive to rise to the top.

My closest friends are hard workers, too. Frankly, they couldn't be my friends if they weren't. I have no time for the lazy. I'm not naive enough to think that hard work equals wealth, nor am I naive enough to think that uneducated or lazy people can't fall into large sums of money by luck, or be born to the lucky sperm club. If we are playing the odds, I would bet on the guy who works hard in his own business.

To make money, the key is, be great at what you do, show enthusiasm, and have a system around you that works. I cannot emphasize this enough. To steal a quote from Warren Buffet, there is no such thing as a good job. Mr. Buffet said that if you want to get rich, quit your job and start creating jobs. I agree! In fact, before I heard Buffet say it, I had already said the same phrase to my friends and colleagues with no idea who Buffet was. That's just the way I was. If you want to win, you have to work hard.

That might not be fair, but is there anyone who thinks we live in a fair society? Boy, are they living under a rock. I have instilled this idea to my children since their respective births: "The only fair thing in life is what you hand the bus driver for entry into the bus. Your fare. Other than that, nothing is fair, and don't expect it to be." My daughter remarked at seven years old that the front of a plane is better than the rear!

Why should anyone think that life should be fair, and that any two people should be equal? Moreover, what kind of a society would we have if that were the case? If everybody looked the same, dressed the same, and spoke the same? There would be no fun to the game of life, and there would be no challenge. This would be a horrible way to live.

Take this story as an example. Say there are ten people in a college class, and it's exam time. One guy studies hard and gets a one hundred. One guy doesn't show up, and the other people all land somewhere in the middle. When it's time to get their grades back, imagine if the teacher just said, "You know what? Everyone gets a seventy." Well, the next time there's a test, many more people are going to stay home. Those who do show up probably won't study first. Since they're all going to end up equal, the upper echelon will never be motivated to do great things, and the lower rungs will never have any hope to rise up. Where's your desire, drive, or inspiration supposed to come from in that case?

If we're all equal, nobody can get ahead. We might as well all give up and fall behind together as a society. I refuse to live that way. From the beginning, I've had my sights set on being better every day.

I might have partied too much in college, though, when my gregarious personality won out over my single-minded focus. I'll let my college roommate, Dave Weksel, explain:

> In college, Steve was the type of guy that didn't get really good grades, but you knew that he was going to be successful. It was

known that he was going down the medical path, that it was his lifelong goal. He was clear that he was going to figure out a way to make it happen even if his grades wouldn't support going to an American med school.

He did obviously study, but he also partook in a lot of social activities. Steve was very successful with the females. That's the goal for a young eighteen-year-old kid when you're living away from home for some period of time, and all the hormones are raging, right? So, we had success there. I would say he was probably an average student as far as grades go, but none of that really mattered. He had goals and you knew he was going to achieve them.

We lived in the same suite with six people: three bedrooms with two kids in each bedroom. We had a common room, and in the common room, we had parties. In fact, Steve's the one who kind of organized the first party we had, he had the "rap."

To have a successful college party, you've got to either have free alcohol or some other draw to get people to come. Steve came up with this great idea: Let's make it "The Legs Party." We were going to have a legs contest and decide who had the nicest legs. I don't remember what the prize was, or if we even had one. That's how we advertised it. In fact, I don't think we gave out a prize after all. I think he made me put up some posters, if I remember correctly, to try to get people to come. Our draw was something unique that no one else came up with. The legs party was brilliant marketing.

We played all sorts of intramural sports together: hockey, football, basketball, and softball. We'd go around the dorm to recruit people to join the teams. The college had this club program where if you had a certain number of people you could get some money and have them pay for your club activities. We tried to do that with weightlifting. So, we got some weights in our room and we would lift weights there. Sometimes, we'd drop them on the floor. The people that lived below us would complain, but we didn't think it was a big deal until the monthly dorm newsletter came out. They wrote that there had been a series of local earthquakes felt in the dorm. I still don't really know if they were joking or serious. Clearly, the weightlifting club didn't really work out, but we ended up being cocaptains of the hockey team together. After the games, we'd go out and hang out together. It was great camaraderie.

We had a great time wherever we went. In the lunchroom, for example, it was very much a free-for-all. Everything from food fights to other kinds of interesting stuff. So, there was a group of guys in a different dorm with whom we had kind of a rivalry. This one time, they were standing at the large bucket of soup, and Steve and I were at a table on the other side of the cafeteria (maybe 100 feet away). These are large cafeterias, but Steve took an apple and threw it all the way across the room. Somehow, it landed into the bucket of soup and splashed all over those guys. We were falling off the chair laughing.

That was the early 1980s, and we've been friends ever since. Steve's the godfather of my kids. I'm godfather to his kids. I was the best man in his wedding. He's given very good guidance to both of my daughters and has a fabulous relationship with my younger daughter, in particular.

My oldest daughter is the same age as his oldest one, and she went into medicine, too. She's entering her first year of residency. He and my daughters, with his son and daughter, all have created a patent related to a new type of hypodermic needle. He started the idea because he's kind of in that space all this time, and I have experience with other patents.

Steve's a wonderful friend, and an extremely loyal person. It takes some time to garner that level of loyalty, but once you're there, it's forever.

My path to success began when I finally started studying medicine in earnest. It truly was my calling.

After graduating Stony Brook, class of 1984, I had a short two months to prepare for what would be the start of a career in medicine, and I wasn't really sure what my next step should be.

My grades weren't the greatest, and my Stony Brook premed advisor wasn't exactly supportive of my dream of being an MD. This is how her "counseling" went:

She told me, "Steve, I'm sorry, but you can't be a doctor. You'll have to try something else."

"Like what?"

"Well . . . you could be a dentist?"

So, I applied to and got into the NYU College of Dentistry, the Temple University School of Dentistry, and the Tufts University School of Dentistry. I didn't move forward with matriculating, though, because I was unenthused.

I met with the advisor again, and I told this lady, "I don't want that. What else could I do?"

She said, "You could be a podiatrist."

Following her advice, I applied and was accepted to the New York Podiatric College of Medicine. Still, it didn't seem right.

Her next genius idea? She asked me, "Why not be a chiropractor?"

So, I applied to and got into New York Chiropractic School. Deep down, I knew that I didn't want to be a chiropractor. The only thing I wanted was to be an MD, and I wouldn't settle for anything else. Still, I was young and naive, so I listened to this stupid woman as she tried to put a cap on my dreams.

At that moment in time, fate intervened. One day, my father came home with a newspaper ad for a Caribbean medical school, the American University of the Caribbean School of Medicine Montserrat British West Indies. With the support of my loving parents, I applied and was accepted in two weeks. (I never applied to a US medical school, in fact.) I was thrilled to be closer to my dream. Screw that advisor. (Stony Brook is now lucky to have the services of James Montren as their director for preprofessional advising. What a great guy and a true asset to the students.)

In September of 1984, my journey began. I flew from New York's JFK airport to Antigua, changed to a puddle jumper, and after a short fifteen-minute flight, I landed in Plymouth on the island of Montserrat.

My arrival wasn't exactly triumphant. It was dark. There was nobody else on the plane, and it looked like the airport was closed. I was nervous. I was alone, and I was definitely far from home. The one bit of connection to my old life—my luggage—could not be found. As I was seriously doubting my decision to go there in the first place, an orange van rolled up, one that could probably fit six or eight people. Somehow, the driver knew me. I didn't know the driver, but I hopped in, and he drove across the island. About ten miles later, he dropped me off at the school—without luggage and with tears in my eyes.

The medical school looked like an old motel and was situated at the base of a volcano—one that would erupt and engulf the entire school roughly ten years later. It seemed deserted, as well. I sat on the steps contemplating my next move in the dark. Out of nowhere a woman came over, and she seemed to know who I was, too. She handed me keys to a dorm room and saw me on my way.

Still with tears in my eyes, and almost two thousand miles from home, I discovered the harsh facts of life. I dried my tears as I found my dorm room and was greeted by a very friendly guy named Rudy, from California. We exchanged pleasantries, and it became clear that Rudy had already been there for a few days, maybe a week. He had already found a network of friends. He was partying; he even had girls in the room. Rudy failed out in two weeks or so.

I was perplexed. I thought I was escaping the party life to begin the imprisoned life of a studyholic. I was on a mission, and failure at this stage was not an option. I'd already tasted failure when I was banished to the Caribbean instead of pursuing a medical career in the US with the rest of my American peers. It had been embarrassing to head off to the Caribbean on my own. The fifty or so premed kids in my college class whom I knew went to medical school in Brooklyn or whatever. Then, another ten went to Guadalajara to take classes in Spanish. A couple went to Europe or elsewhere, and then I and a few others went to the Caribbean. We were seen as the bottom of the barrel.

At the same time, I knew that the route I was taking could end up in the same place if I stayed the course. My "never say no" attitude took over as I made peace with the imprisonment of studying and eating USDA Grade C food! (Sorry, can't make this up.) I became a library recluse for the greater part of four-and-a-half semesters and walked with a pipe to fight off stray dogs that didn't like the Grade C chicken, either. We had the SAC-student activity center, where married student spouses made baked goods. Any home food we brought was stolen by the local airport rogue customs officers.

Whatever you may think—and no matter what I thought before going there—Caribbean med school is no joke. The curriculum on the island of Montserrat ("the rock," as we called it) included the exact same courses, textbooks, and actual professors from the American medical schools. No joke, I took twenty-four credits one semester. These professors were great across the board. Some came down for a semester at a time on sabbatical to teach us medical students, and others would come down to teach for years after ending their careers in the US or Britain. No matter how long they were there for, they would teach with a passion. They knew that anybody who would travel to the Caribbean to become a doctor back in the United States must have heart, and that was true, for one-third of us. We were up against a lot, but some of us were determined to make it through.

Day to day, it didn't always feel like a sure thing. Rumors came and rumors went that the school was closing, or worse. It felt like something bad was always happening, or about to happen.

On at least one occasion, it did. The most memorable of my experiences on the island was living through a 7.7 earthquake on the Richter scale (an OMG moment). My first earthquake was so much fun. I had never seen or felt anything like it growing up in the Northeast, unlike students from the West Coast. I was dumbstruck as I sat at my desk and watched the ceiling shake above me and felt the concrete rumble below me. Students dived under the desks or fled to the doorways. Upon standing, I was knocked over by a wave—one that appeared to be an ocean wave but was in fact concrete. Literally, a three-foot wave of concrete knocked everyone standing in the room off their feet. For six months I maintained a low-grade headache and dizzy feeling—such pleasure.

Fortunately, there were no tall buildings in the area, and fortunately nobody got hurt. At the end of it all, however, it looked like somebody had taken a butter knife and cut the island by about ten meters all around. Aftermath shocks rocked the island for months, sometimes up to 4.0. We were like a rowboat in the ocean.

(It wouldn't be the last natural disaster to strike the region. Later, the poor island became victim to Hurricane Hugo and the eruption of the volcano Mount Soufrière, which completely demolished the city of Plymouth and my old medical school. Today, it lies in a Pompeii-like field of ash and for the most part remains off limits to guests or returning students. However, knowing some of the old locals goes a long way in getting a sneak peek at the off-limits areas.)

The earthquake never shook my purpose. However, my mother was nervous. For the next six months, she was on the phone with the seismic center in Colorado all day long, making sure there was no tidal wave coming to wash her son away from the Caribbean. Mom and dad were very concerned for my well-being at all times, as I was an only child. She begged me to come home, but I would not listen to any of her exhortations. My goal was to become a physician, an MD, and to be able to practice wherever I chose in the United States. Eventually, my parents got the picture. They said to stop listening to the rumors, to just buckle down and study. Mom said go where you will achieve the best and one day dad and I will go there; ironically, as they have aged, that is exactly what occurred. They would try to keep track of any looming disasters at the school, or anything else they could figure out.

Soon, however, I'd be leaving Montserrat to fly across the pond, as I spent my third and part of my fourth year of medical school in London. Even now, I still say that no part of my life could be better. After all of those months studying in the Caribbean, I was ready to let loose.

It felt like destiny when I met Robert Feferman on the airplane on the way to London. We got off the plane, looked at each other, and said, "We need to get an apartment together." So, we found a house and two other guys to share it with. One guy was a Mormon (he left his wife and kids in Utah and had tons of fun in London), and the other guy was a former CIA agent who had the posture of a giraffe and a rhinoceros put together—he wasn't much fun. He was way more than twenty years our senior, and the medicine thing was clearly a second career for him. Anyway, this guy would lock himself in his room, and I don't know what the hell he would do. I think he had a coffeepot in his room, and he would just stay there getting caffeinated.

Meanwhile, Rob and I were on the loose. Our parents were on the other side of the ocean. We didn't have anyone to answer to. We didn't have anyone to ask us if we did our homework. We didn't have anyone to tell us when to go to bed or when to wake up. Just like carrying a machete or a gun on a plane would probably land you in Sing Sing today, everything we did in London is probably now a felony. (By the way, I did carry a gun on a plane in the seventies, when flying home from a summer job. A guy had given me a Saturday night special on the job and I thought it was cool. In March of '86, I flew home from Montserrat with one machete in my carry-on and one in my fist. Let's just say, carry-on rules have changed a lot over the last few decades.)

We were running amok, having parties was ubiquitous, picking up girls left and right. Rob and I had immense fun (we found ataraxia). We took the tube to the Hippodrome and Stringfellows every weekend. I was filling my black book, sowing my oats without any parental supervision. At the same time, I did keep my neighbor as my "girlfriend" the whole time I lived there. Her mom cooked me Sunday dinner every weekend. I learned about bubble and squeak, bangers, and toad in the hole, it was perfect. My mom really thought I would just get married and never come back.

Here's Rob with an inside take on all the mischief we got up to:

Steve and I met in London, about 1985. We both went to the same school in the Caribbean, and we both ended up doing our clinical rotations at the same hospital in London. Our personalities just clicked.

He definitely has an outgoing personality. He's really open and flirtatious. On the other hand, he was always the smartest one in the group. I mean, whether people liked him or not, he was always the guy who knew the answer to every question that some doctors would ask.

This was right back when AIDS was starting, and we were sitting in some lecture when we heard the word AIDS for the first time. We didn't even know what it was. The lights were out, and they were showing the pathology slides, showing these cells. Finally, Steve says, those are foam cells. Everyone was like, what? He picked it up when most of us—including the doctors in the room—hadn't even heard of it. It was like he'd already been studying it for months. I was like, how the hell does anyone know that?

He always seemed a little more motivated and disciplined than everyone else. He'd spend a couple days in his room, just reading, and then hit the pubs when he came out. He studied hard and he played hard.

Subway Soloway. That was my nickname for him in London. Every time we rode on that stupid subway, he met like twenty people. *We* couldn't walk down the street without him having to talk to somebody. Most of the time, it was a girl.

Steve went out with hundreds of girls, and I'm not exaggerating. He always had a couple of girlfriends, and he was always meeting a girl every time he went somewhere. It was all like clockwork: Steve would hit on a girl right up front, so she'd either like him or leave. Most of the time, they liked him. WE were popular for some reason to those British girls. They loved our accent. We were Teflon. Steve flipped when he was called a bloke; we had never heard the term and thought it was derogatory, only to find out it meant "a guy."

He actually had a book where he wrote down all his girlfriends and took pictures of them. He always kept tabs.

To this day, his passion for life has not dwindled. He travels more now than ever, and he's busier than anyone I know. I don't know how he does what he does, and I know he doesn't do drugs. You would think he did speed or something, but he's naturally high like that.

You would never think he'd become a doctor, because he was such a wild ass, but he still is one today. *Any* crazy stories he tells you are true. That's all that I can say. (Dr. Chen said you must work hard and play hard, but "you must get laid on Friday night." Dr. Chen was our anesthesia professor and could not be distracted from a crossword puzzle during anesthesia, ever!) Chen taught us "blind intubation." If you put the tube through the nose and hoped it went in the trachea, not the esophagus. He called it repeatedly "blind intubation, since you can't see" in his thick Chinese accent. Oh the memories! Mr. Baldwin, our gynecology professor, made us learn vaginal exams. He emphasized the importance, and he made us stick two fingers in every vagina in the clinic for hours at a time; he was very prolific. In fact, a total hysterectomy was twelve minutes skin to skin. And by the way, the surgeons there and here compete like that. Watch out who does your hysterectomy! We were taught that any patient entering the hospital gets a rectal exam: "The only reason for no exam is no finger or no asshole."

One of my other London roommates, Kurt Henry, wanted to add his take: "Some of us should be banned from going back to London."

I played hard but studied hard, too. It's not bragging to say you're the superstar of the Caribbean med school kids. Always following other doctors around until they were tired of seeing my face, learning, watching, and doing. While my college friends were in medical school in Brooklyn, reading books, I obtained invaluable hands-on education. We were taking out appendixes and gallbladders, putting down ET tubes, starting triple lumen catheters, Foley catheters, arterial blood gasses, and lumbar punctures. This was third-year medical school. None of my friends from college had ever done anything like it at that level. It would take them years, even decades, before they achieved the skills I adroitly mastered in London.

One of the more exciting examples of a hands-on task came during my obstetric rotation: I got to deliver twins. Delivering twins in the United States would not be possible for a medical student. It would be reserved for only the most elite fellows, perhaps even an Ivy Leaguer specializing in high-risk pregnancies. Yet there I was, a twenty-three-year-old medical student delivering twins, performing C-sections, executing episiotomies (they said suture in layers, which I had not heard prior to this!), and basically doing everything that the attending physicians were doing. That hands-on experience probably reflects in my career today. I have not run into too many people with the wide range of hands-on practical skills that I have—other than the people that I trained with in the Caribbean.

One night in the emergency department in Kingston Hospital, the senior doctors asked me to see a patient after hours. I approached the patient, and after 30 or 45 minutes of trying to have a conversation, I walked out of the room shaking my head and had no idea what was going on. I could not get an answer to any question that made any sense at all, yet the patient seemed to take it all in stride. As I left the room, all the seniors were laughing hysterically to tell me that this was a confabulating alcoholic. Another adventure was my psychiatry rotation—the scary locked prison ward for sociopaths (serious fear), and the group meetings for patients that would stand and urinate on the table, or "the ice skater" as I labeled a woman who walked the halls with a hand behind her back and her tongue glued to the wall, hours on end, day after day. I recall standing at a bedside with a professor and three or five students. The patient had jaundice, we discussed jaundice and its causes for hours, I don't think the patient was aware he had jaundice.

Everything in that program was teaching-oriented. I remember being called up in an audience of hundreds of people for a special lecture—like our "grand rounds." They had this person sitting on the stage. They would tell you one or two of the person's symptoms, and you had to diagnose what was wrong with them. They only picked very rare and unusual stuff. It was like a live episode of *House*.

Somehow—I don't know why or how—I got called up there out of all the students and all the trainees in all of the hospital.

They tell me, "Here's this person sitting in a chair," and right away I noticed the person's legs. The rash was typical, what we call palpable purpura. It was like small red dots that are slightly elevated. I would say you need to have experienced or have at least seen it and touched it once to know it again. At the time, I really had such a small point of knowledge that I didn't know a lot of things that could do that. I knew what it was right away, but I didn't say anything.

They said to me, "Okay, we're going to tell you one other thing about this person," as I'm sitting there like an idiot.

I said nothing.

They said something like, "His platelet count is normal. So, what do you want to know next? What are your thoughts and what do you think? Do you have questions for the patient?

I said, "Oh yes. It's Henoch-Schoenlein purpura." I swear to God, for the next thirty seconds you could hear a pin drop. It was like I was Dr. House, like no one else could have solved it. No one else had a clue. (Ironically, it's now called IGA vasculitis, and I see it all the time!)

During that period of my life, I was like a sponge, following around the doctors like a puppy; in fact, I never thought I knew enough and stayed late many nights begging to learn about every admission. In England, they were called registrars or senior registrars, in contradistinction to interns or residents, as we call them in the US. The language of medicine was slightly different from in the US, but we fit right in. We learned IVs, intubation. We learned how to resuscitate. We learned how to practice medicine. We could talk to patients, take histories. We were on top of the world. We thought we knew it all, and for where we were in the world at that time, we probably did.

As students, we had true white-coat rounds. We would gather around the bedside with an esteemed professor, and with permission from the patients. We had a human textbook at our disposal on a regular basis both for history taking and physical exam findings and learning about disease processes. Many of the cases I saw then, more than 30 years ago, have stuck with me.

Finally, I graduated in the upper echelon of my class. My class had been the largest starting classes that the school had ever had, with more than two hundred students. (Granted, the school had only been open for six years, but anyway. . . .) Of those, only about seventy ended up becoming physicians at the end. Many people left for various reasons. Some left quickly, and others stuck it out for years trying and failing to pass the exam needed to come back to the United States and formally practice medicine. Some came because tuition was cheaper than vacation!

Those board exams were originally called ECFMG certificates (Educational Commission on Foreign Medical School Graduates), but in my days they were called FMGEMS, or Foreign Medical Graduate Examination in the Medical Sciences. This was the same exam given under the name of the US national medical board exam. The only difference was, if you went to school in the United States, you needed to be in the bottom two standard deviations to pass the exam. If you were a Caribbean or international student, you needed to be in the top two. The FMGEM was meant to weed out international med school grads who couldn't cut it. If you read carefully, we as foreign grads were held to a higher academic standard then USA graduates!

Getting a seventy-five equated to landing in the top two standard deviations. I passed with an eighty-one, so I must've been four standard deviations above the mean. I don't think I even heard of two people who got more than that. That was about as high as you could get, but it's not like I got a gold star or anything. There was so much discrimination that went into effect back then to keep out foreign medical grads. By all rights, any medical grad in the eighties who passed the FMGEM exam was by definition in the upper echelon of all US medical students across the board—everywhere from Harvard to Howard, with no exceptions. That group included me.

My time in Montserrat and in London had made me more convinced than ever that I was destined to become an MD. Other lessons I learned along the way were just as vital. Through the years living out of the country forming groups for studying and socializing, I formed lifelong bonds. This camaraderie among colleagues became a lifelong habit that never died.

The next chapter in my medical career was that of internship and residency. Of course, brainwashed and naive, I was again convinced that I was not worthy of going to a major university residency program. That was in no small part thanks to the famous gastroenterologist Dr. Jay Thomas Lamont.

Before graduation and after London, I finished my fourth year of medical school by doing rotations in the United States. I did three months in Omaha, Nebraska, at Creighton University, and that was followed by three months at Boston University. One in particular was in Boston University gastroenterology with Dr. Lamont, an author of Harrison's textbook, *The Principles of Internal Medicine*.

Dr. Lamont was the most famous GI guy in the world at the time. He clearly thought he was the smartest guy in the room—and he was on GI issues, but personal skills were far below that of someone living under a mushroom. The truth is, I was intimidated by him, and rather than encourage me, he shot me down. The other truth was his personality was so bad he was probably forced into academic medicine and could never be in his own practice.

I first encountered Dr. Lamont on a rotation, fresh off my stint in London and flying high. After a small miscommunication due to the difference between the UK and US systems, Dr. Lamont told me that I should probably think about another career. I knew his field of knowledge was narrow, but still, his words hurt me—they stunted my progress. Instead of aiming high for my next step, I took a residency at a community hospital system (rather than a university teaching hospital system) called Mercy Catholic Medical Center. There were two divisions: one in West Philadelphia, Misericordia, and the other on the outskirts of Philadelphia, Fitzgerald Mercy Hospital. In the end, though, that would turn out to be a blessing.

The composition of the community hospital's patients was split into two divisions: an urban knife-and-gun club, and a lower-middle-class mixed ethnic group. My trial by fire began in early July 1988.

Coincidentally, one of my fellow Caribbean med school grads and former London roomie, Kurt Henry, ended up there doing his residency, too. Here's how Kurt describes the scene:

> Misericordia was where they dropped the infamous bomb. In 1985, the offices of the black liberation group MOVE were bombed. Well, guess what. Our hospital was across the street. There was a lot of hostility in the area. At the same time, the City of Philadelphia had filed for bankruptcy, and medical care got cut. It was the interns and residents that ran that hospital. We did everything, for about $21,958 a year.
>
> We came in and we saw the fraud. We saw the abuse. We saw people doing drugs on the job. Surgeons operating drunk—this is no joke. This is serious. We learned the dark side of medicine. The Hippocratic Oath got thrown out so many times, it was ridiculous.
>
> There was a surgical resident who looked down on us because we were Caribbean med school grads. He was a total asshole: racist, anti-Semitic, and prejudiced. I remember I was taking care of an AIDS patient who was on a ventilator, treating him aggressively to knock him down with morphine and Ativan, and nothing was working. I was at his bedside all through the night into the morning for this guy, who ended up dying. That resident was a total dick about it and gave me a hard time about not being able to get him

down. Weeks later, I found out why my drug wasn't working: One of the nurses was signing off for the drugs and replacing them with saline. She was injecting herself in the nurse's room with the drugs that we were prescribing to the patient. Patients were treated so poorly at times. I recall Steve needing to write for the nurses to change bed sheets and clean ice cubes off a bed from an intensive care patient.

In that broken system, Steve still managed to excel. You could really see his development begin to take off.

I was learning a lot, but it turned out that it still wasn't enough. I'll never forget when I was on call for one of the first times in my life. Shortly after call started, I was fighting with my beeper, getting calls constantly. One in particular was from a nurse by the name of Cara, calling me to the telemetry unit at Misericordia Hospital for a patient with shortness of breath. I believe I was watching TV in the resident's lounge on the sixth floor when this call came.

I ran down three flights of stairs to the scene. In spite of the fact that it was my very first day, I was on the case. It was the first time I was faced with the harsh reality of medical care: Protocol always wins out over patients. Patients always come last, never forget that. Nurse Cara had called me for a patient who had shortness of breath and was partially in shock. (I was partially in shock, because I didn't know what to do!)

She immediately said to me, "Doc, order a chest X-ray. Order a blood gas. Check the pulse. Ask for the chart." Cara went through everything with me. It was obvious that Cara knew far more about how to take care of that patient on that day then I ever could have. Cara had done this for many years and had seen many neophytes before me. She helped me get through that night. But Cara lit a fire under me that never stopped burning.

I took my Washington Manual, I ran to my room, and I immediately read every chapter on shortness of breath. I immediately started reading about heart failure, pneumonia, pneumothorax, pulmonary embolism. I started reading about atrial fibrillation, ventricular dysrhythmias, sepsis. I think I covered the whole book in five minutes. I was a neophyte, but I grew up that night. From that point forward, I welcomed calls for shortness of breath. In fact, within months, I was involved in dozens of codes: resuscitation of dead people in all aspects, including the intubation, chest compressions, barking out orders to push medications, starting sophisticated central lines, and on occasion a chest tube. I felt like I owned the hospital at that point; the learning curve was 0–60 in less than one second. This learning curve was not for all. It was only for those who were highly motivated and willing to put in the work and effort.

Before long, camaraderie set in. We were all in the same boat. Nobody knew what was going on, but we all learned from one another. Typically, we were organized in groups with two residents, one third year, one second year, and two or three interns. We walked around together, and we learned together. We took emergency calls together. We taught one another.

Typically, we were on call every fourth night, and back then you did most of your learning at night. That said, if you add in all the moonlighting, we were sleeping at the hospital every two or three nights. In a typical "day," you worked from 9:00 a.m. to 5:00 p.m., and then at 5:00 p.m., you had sign-outs. You would receive sign-out rounds from the ICU and the other monitored beds for the sickest people. That meant that you'd go to the cafeteria to meet with the physicians from the ICU to learn about their patients. If they needed help during the night, we would need to know everything we should about them. While we were parenthetically guarding those sick patients, we were being called to other floors: sometimes for Tylenol orders, sleeping pills, procedures that needed to be done, people needing to urinate, catheters needing to be placed. Sometimes people could not move their bowels, and we had to manually disimpact them. Occasionally an emergency would hit the ER, and we would have to run down and stop what we were doing. A situation like that would take precedence over the old man who could not pee.

Gunshot victims were common. But so was asthma, heart attacks, GI bleeds, psychotic events, meningitis, pneumonia, burn victims, and anything you can imagine! I even diagnosed tsutsugamushi fever. Working in the emergency rooms was not always safe. I recall one occasion when a patient grabbed a knife or scalpel and was acting crazy—threatening and trying to stab anybody within his reach. Fortunately, security was numerous and plentiful. They were able to subdue him with nobody injured. I recall leaving the scene with the head of security. He showed me his desk—he had confiscated nearly fifty kitchen knives from people entering the emergency room doors over a three-month period of time. We were placing chest tubes, endotracheal tubes, catheters in both upper and both lower extremities, running fluid as fast as possible, typing and cross-matching blood as fast as possible to find out which blood was safe to give to which patient. We inserted pacemakers, Swan-Ganz catheters, did open cardiac massage, and did fluid and ventilator management ourselves. At night there are no attendings! We were amazing at saving lives when it came to people who were either passed out, shot, unconscious, or otherwise not living when they came to the emergency room. It became second nature.

It was so common that if an unconscious person came in and there was no obvious injury, they would receive a cocktail in case they were drunk, vitamin-deficient, or overdosed. After years of doing it, I found the emergencies all to be the same. Whether a patient was short of breath, their heart stopped, or they were bleeding to death, the end results were always the same: IV fluids, ACLS protocol, CPR, mechanical ventilation, pressers, and a lot of prayer.

We became comfortable with dead bodies and desensitized to the concept of death. It was likely easier to deal with being an indestructible twentysomething. If it were to happen all over again later in life, I do not know if I could have taken it in stride so easily. It wasn't a lack of caring, however. Whether it was because of the system or the surrounding neighborhood, death just seemed to be commonplace. We didn't stop to mourn. More important, we had clinics to run.

In one typical example, I remember an episode where a patient came to the clinic with a penile wart. I was told to remove it, even though I had never used the equipment before and didn't't know what to do. I had never even seen this equipment, which was called a Bovie machine. I kept telling the attending physician at the clinic that I had no hands-on experience and I shouldn't't do it, but he wasn't't swayed. I was told that it was "See one, do one, teach one," and if I hadn't seen one, I should pretend that I had seen one and just do it. So, I went in blind and tackled that man's penis. I injected Lidocaine into the wart and just burned the shit out of it. I don't know if he ever healed, but that wart definitely will never come back. (All these years later, I feel dreadfully sorry for that man.)

In addition to the general clinic, there was a hematology/oncology clinic for uninsured patients. Because I was ambitious, I was selected to run it. In essence, I was the hematologist/oncologist for the uninsured people. I was making the decisions, leading as I went. The backup was a family practitioner, who would always encourage me to just go ahead and do it if it made sense at the time. This position even led to me doing in-house moonlighting on the cancer floor of the hospital. At this stage of my career, I had seen and/or cared for each of the nine varieties of acute myelogenous leukemia. This is unheard of in today's world.

Was I overambitious? Not necessarily. I was following instructions, and I was young. I truly listen and learn when I am the student, and I am truly obedient to authority. No one stopped me, and above all, I was there to learn. Indeed, I did learn one of the most brutal lessons I would ever learn about our system: hospitals aren't necessarily there to help people get better. (Basically, you never want to be a patient.)

It took me a long time to understand that when people got sick in the hospital, they nearly always died. I was still in my early twenties, but I could see that people from age fifty on up would come in, and often they would never get out. It could have been pneumonia, asthma, GI bleed; it could have been most anything. In nearly every case, it would be fatal. I never knew if it was because they had come from a bad neighborhood, or if it was because sepsis would often set in. Often, I wondered if they'd have been better off not coming to the hospital in the first place.

They might not have even really needed to be there. At times, we were pressured to fill beds at any cost. If the hospital census was low, the hospital administration would tell us how many people to admit. They always wanted all the beds filled.

The stream of patients was endless. Back then we had many AIDS patients, infections, many strokes, overdoses, many episodes of trauma. I recall one man who had set his own brother on fire with gasoline—on the emergency room doorstep, on the Fourth of July. I recall treating a patient who was smoking a cigarette in an oxygen mask, which caused the patient's face to explode. Once, I set a chest tube and subsequently got my entire body drenched in blood. (It was during the early days of the AIDS epidemic, and I must have spent hours in the shower after, scrubbing myself and crying over the thought that I'd "caught" AIDS.) There were many stories, but the final outcome was typically the same: the person usually perished.

In some ways, I started to become numb. Frankly, there wasn't really anybody there to make sure people were getting saved. They only cared that you showed up for work and presented the projects or assignments that were given to you.

Of course, at the end of the day you needed to be prepared to pass the boards. Not passing the boards would reflect poorly upon the program, and they would lose money. With loss of money would come fewer residency spots. The typical arrangement is that the federal government gives hospitals money for teaching, while hospitals pay the residents half in salary and keep the rest for the administration. That is just one of the highly dysfunctional systems in our country.

Ironically, nobody ever really taught rheumatology specifically, but over time I realized that anything interesting I saw seemed to be related to rheumatology. After the second year of my residency, Dr. Tony Albornoz became chair of the department, and he was a rheumatologist. He often would point out the most interesting cases, which were always in rheumatology. I found it absolutely fantastic. Rheumatology always involved the things we'd never heard of. There was nothing about cardiology, pulmonary, kidney, or GI that was interesting to me. We were doing that all day and all night, almost 365 days a year. When something different happened, it was interesting, and it was often rheumatological.

For patients, we say it is never good to be an interesting case because if you are interesting, it means nobody knows what is wrong, or what to do with you. With every case, though, I tried to learn as I went along and tried to do my best to help people. In good conscience, I tried to uphold the Hippocratic Oath—at least, the part about doing no intentional harm.

That wasn't the case with everyone. We had some shady characters in our program. I am referring to the teaching staff and attending physicians, and some students and residents. Some, rather than writing and completing charts, would literally take charts by the hundreds and just put them out in the trash, so they didn't have to deal with them. We had doctors who would sit at a desk at the nurse's station and call each patient's room. They'd ask if the patient was there, and upon hearing the patient's voice, they'd write a note in the chart that the patient was fine. They told the nurses to call them later if there were any issues. It was such a dereliction of duty—if it wasn't criminal! Another attending would walk in the room and grab the patient's chart. He'd write on every chart, "As above, see below. If you need me, let me know," and he'd go home.

We also had residents—some of whom spoke very broken English and didn't follow directions—who insisted on doing procedures with no supervision. On several occasions, they would be caught threading guidewires while putting in an IV line, and wires were lost. Patients were rushed to emergency interventional radiology, so they could find the wire that had been lost. Rather than cutting them open, they put them under a fluoroscope, put some forceps in the vessel, and pulled the wire out. It was a big ordeal, and all because the community hospital had a coterie of non-English-speaking doctors who didn't stop to ask questions.

Operating room patients were dropped on the floor while surgeons chuckled over their weight. I previously noted that some surgeons have been witnessed operating intoxicated. Women would show up (on purpose) at three in the morning asking for vaginal exams. The doctor would put on mirrored sunglasses because he thought it was all just a joke. Some of the pregnant patients were so young, they didn't know if they were sexually active—or even what that meant. One girl asked me, "How would I know if I'm sexually active if I don't watch?" Others would come in filled with used condoms and swear that they had never had sex. It was incredibly heartbreaking.

We saw a man with back pain. Nobody knew why, until he took his coat off and we saw that he had a bullet through his coat and in his back. He couldn't understand how or why this happened. I saw another man show up in the emergency room with something in his hand due to a large hernia. The object was his stomach.

Patients often became violent, either from drugs or coming off of drugs. At our hospital, we had four-point leather restraints; at others, they had five, including the neck with the strap to the floor. They were all given as much Haldol as they could take without dying, and they were secured to the floor by their extremities and thick leather shackles. Oftentimes, they would sleep it off; often they would not wake up at all. It was all part of the job. Still, the program needed to go on, as all programs at hospitals need money to run. (A note about the system: we were told to admit or not admit patients based on the census and cash flow needs of the system.)

As I moved on to my fellowship, it became more interesting. At that time, they placed American medical students first. As an international or foreign medical graduate, I was limited, or at least thought I was limited, to sub-specialties within internal medicine. We were the lowest pieces of mold on the totem pole, but it all worked out for me.

I really did enjoy it. I found that rheumatology was a bit of a specialty for a gentleman, a thinking man's art, like a chess game. What came as a shock to me, however, was the fact that a good rheumatologist is an orthopedic surgeon without a knife—and by far, a better craftsman with a needle. When it comes to *good* rheumatologists, though, there aren't many. (Most orthopedic surgeons do everything better than most rheumatologists today, but I'm not most rheumatologists.) In fact, from my first needling of a joint to the most recent one thirty years later, I have never met a patient who had a better experience with an orthopedic surgeon than they had with me. Not one, not yet, not ever. Still, the orthopedic doctors always acted like they were entitled. (I must share a secret: When I was a medical student in London and one of the attending physicians ordered me to draw up Lidocaine, I did not know what he meant. I did not know what to do, and I ended up breaking the glass vial—a single use vial—in my hand, cutting myself, and the Lidocaine spilled all over the floor.)

Dermatologists were the most elite, It was virtually impossible to get a spot in that field, and they made sure you knew it. When I spent my time at Boston City Hospital doing dermatology as an elective before my residency, there were three fellowship spots. One was taken by a valedictorian from an Ivy League medical school; another was a Middle Easterner whose family donated ten million dollars to the department. I cannot recall the third person, but I am certain that he or she did not graduate from a Caribbean medical school.

I was an outlier in every sense, I conformed to my rules, and that shaped my path. I am better for it. Even though the neighborhoods were dangerous, the pay was low, and there was racism, discrimination, and bad care running rampant, I am grateful for my time at Misericordia. In fact, I have found that the best-trained doctors—in spite of everything—usually were trained at community hospitals. I believe this is just one reason why I am the best.

Anyway, after Misericordia, it was time to get to work. I had a rheumatology fellowship at the Medical College of Pennsylvania—two years learning everything I could about rheumatology. In fact, during my training, I worked at night in a private rheumatology practice. That physician and I are still friends today. He told me I taught him a lot. I joke with him that letting me go was the worst mistake he ever made. He agrees. Thank you, Barry Getzoff. I went up and down through Pennsylvania, Northern Delaware, and the entire state of New Jersey in search of a job. After interviewing in five or ten offices, I quickly decided that working for somebody else was not for me. It wasn't that the money wasn't good. The offers for starting salaries ranged from $55,000 to $90,000 per year, and back then, $40,000 to $50,000 sounded like a fortune! In fact, when I graduated college, my roommates and I felt if we could make $100,000 a year, we would be the richest people on the planet. We had absolutely no conception of money.

I wasn't blinded by those dollar signs, though. When I finally looked around at all the doctors in all the practices and hospitals and centers in the United States, I decided that the self-employment route was the only one that suited my needs. Why should I listen to somebody else? Why should I walk around, scheduled at all hours, when I could set my own hours? Why on Earth would I want to share the profits with somebody else, when I was the one doing all the work?

That said, I knew from the beginning that I must hire great staff and take care of them. This is mandatory and not easy to find. You find out who your best staff members are, and you treat them like family. In fact, if you can form a good family, they can last forever. They can all be happy. They can all feed their families. They can all take vacations. They can even be proud of the boss. They can be happy with the boss. They can show enthusiasm when the boss does great things. It becomes a great experience—a community instead of just a job.

That is what I undertook in July 1993, renting space for my office in the small town of Vineland, New Jersey—by myself, knowing full well there was no other rheum doc for forty miles. At that time, I made my decision to go to Cumberland County, which is quite a large county. Although people do not know the major city in Cumberland County, which is Vineland, it was once the auxiliary capital of the state at the time of World War II. It's actually the largest city by land in New Jersey. This city, predominantly lower-middle class, seemed to have something unique about it. It had the most profitable fast-food chains in the country. It had the most profitable pharmacies in the country. It had the most profitable liquor stores, convenience stores, and motels in the country. What was it about this town in New Jersey that seemed to have just the right mix of people?

When I first applied for hospital privileges back in 1993, the requirement was that you had to live within five to ten miles of the hospital. There were no exceptions. By today's standards, this is ludicrous, but back then, it seemed to be in the culture. It was not necessarily a bad culture. There were some pros and cons. Regardless, it was because of this requirement that I moved to Vineland.

In Vineland, it seemed as though literally everybody were related to somebody, so I had to be very careful whom I befriended and whom I insulted. I kept my guard up at all times, not knowing who was really a friend, and who was not. There were those who tried to offer assistance because I was the new doctor in town. The local synagogue tried to offer me new business to join up, for example. There also were those who told me point-blank, "We don't have arthritis in this part of the country, you need to go back to the city where you came from." People even threatened me: "If you're friends with doctors we don't like, we're going to run you out of town." One big fat cardiologist said to me 27 years ago, "Leave town, you won't make it." I wish him the best as he is smiling up at the daisies. Those people inspired me to do more.

I did know of an old-timer within my field with a good reputation who would spend about one day per month in the county, but nobody before me was full-time in Cumberland or Salem County. Frankly, at the time of this writing, that is still true. (I do have an associate and have had nurse practitioners, and physician assistants.)

However, I didn't get to where I am today just by picking the right place to start my practice. How does one really reach to the sky and reach to the top? Well, you do need staff, you do need some knowledge, and you certainly need a good personality. You have to make the patients feel at home, and you need to be a chameleon. You have to assume the personality and the accent of the person in front of you at every given visit. In effect, you are an actor playing the role of a different person, male or female, in every act—each act being a visit. Once the patient feels that you are equal to them and truly can understand their complaints and problems, in most cases you have a friend for life. And once again I cannot reemphasize one must work very hard and for long hours using laser focus and not get distracted. One must continue honing their skills, reading articles and journals, attending review courses and other educational activities. Retrospectively, I say a subspecialist needs at least seven years in practice before they can actually know they're good at what they do.

After a period of time, you are still not a well-seasoned doctor, but you have a lot of people believing in you. That is when the barter system starts. You start getting farmers bringing apples, pears, peaches, strawberries, blueberries, corn, onions, potatoes, pigs, cow, sides of beef, entire animals. Handymen, tree cutters, lawn men offering their services. In fact, I started to feel like a politician! All I had to do was go to work, and if I helped people, nobody in the county would take my money: not the local restaurant, not the local workers. Because if I helped somebody get out of pain, or diagnosed the arthritis that they had lived with for a long time, all of a sudden, I was part of the family. Over time, this family grew and grew.

After about seven years in practice, the family grew so much that I had no more room. It was time to upgrade. I had amassed enough money to achieve my short-term dream, which was to buy my own office. For those in business—or even not in business—you know that the most important real estate you will ever own is the real estate that you lease to yourself and invest in for yourself. I was proud to have achieved that milestone—one that I would repeat many times.

This process continued every few years until I was capable of expanding my office to a comprehensive arthritis service center. By encompassing all necessary services within my field in one location, I was able to achieve better patient compliance, which ultimately leads to better patient care and keeps people from becoming hospitalized patients, as there was no room for falling through the cracks. If we wanted a patient to get a CAT scan, X-rays, DXA, blood tests, microscopic evaluation of synovial fluid, or anything else, it was all there. The patients like this model very much.

That system created a sort of convenience never seen before: not by physicians in other states or big cities, not by any of the locals, not even by my parents, who are my biggest fans from day one and continue to be my biggest fans.

Zia Golestaneh watched me create this empire from the beginning:

> Dr. Soloway and I met about twenty-six-and-a-half years ago. He
> was new in his office, and my billing office was next door to him.
> It quickly became clear that he is a genius, and whatever he touches
> turns to gold.
>
> I watched him build that practice from zero to the biggest prac-
> tice I have ever seen, and I have worked for the hospital. Every day,
> maybe sixty to seventy patients come in from all over: New Jersey,
> Pennsylvania, Baltimore, you name it.
>
> Beyond his natural talents, he's very up-to-date. He reads a lot.
> He goes to conferences a lot. I've never seen anybody that dedi-
> cated. Once I said, "What are you going to do this weekend?" and
> he said, "I'm going to Los Angeles." He went there for two days and
> came back Monday night. No hesitation. He goes to Moscow for
> four days and comes right back into work. It's endless energy.
>
> I personally had pain in my hand, my shoulder joint, my hip,
> and a trigger finger, and he injected them. An orthopod had
> missed it, but he figured out what was going on.
>
> At this point, he doesn't need the money. He's working for the
> fun of it. He really loves helping people.

And what fun it is. Any dreams that my parents had for me, any hopes that
I had for myself, my wildest imaginings were soon far surpassed as I rose
almost to the level of celebrity status in my field.

Indeed, over the years, celebrities, dignitaries, and professional athletes
and team owners from many sports have passed through my doors or have
had me fly out to them to do an on-call. Some offer this information publicly
on social media and like to brag for me, while others like to keep a low pro-
file. Over time, I found that there was no amount of money that could ever
equal the connection that was made by helping somebody—either by saving
their life or by eliminating their pain, or both. This was an epiphenomenon

that I never thought or dreamed of as reality. It was experience learned on the fly.

The other leverage I discovered was in my interactions with insurance companies. When the insurance companies realized everything was done within one location, all of a sudden, they were impressed with the concept, because they hadn't seen anyone ever make a medical center, more than just an office, like I had done. Why should they have people who would otherwise be noncompliant (and cost them more money by needing hospitalization) when they could come to my office and have all their X-rays and all other testing or administration of medication done in one place? I've been able to save them money by keeping people compliant and out of the hospital. However, insurance companies have become parsimonious. I will share a heated letter I wrote to an insurance company in support of a patient. This is one of many I've had to write:

October 31, 2019

Dear Sonya "P,"

You have written an incoherent letter addressed to me, on October 2, 2019. This disingenuous letter is to notify me of a nonpayment of services rendered in May of 2019.

I am the patient, why would you notify me six (6) months later, are you short of staff or brains? Why would I, as the patient, receive this? I am the patient and followed my doctor's orders as advised.

While no one with a fruitful day will recall what test occurred six months ago, I suspect this was a 4D-CT Scan, which, was ordered by Dr. Ausiello, an endocrinologist, at Columbia University in New York City. How dubious of you to presume I have my own medical history or records. It's people like yourself that have no knowledge base and make unfounded determinations. I advise you to make appropriate requisitions and handle this yourself. Whatever you denied is without basis (not that you would understand).

I pay $4,000.00 monthly for health insurance, and if things are not taken care of properly, I will hold you in obstruction of proper care. Guidelines are for the impoverished minds (like yours) but are not rules or laws. No hard worker leaves their own businesses to waste time driving one-plus hours to get testing and to lose business.

Furthermore, the test ordered is not listed. How can someone dispute NOTHING? This is a very nefarious system. I hope you further your education, and God Bless You.

Over the years, I've performed millions (literally) of injections/needling procedures. Nobody can believe it until they see me in action. I'm a machine. *I'm the one-man gang. (There was a pro wrestler with the pseudonym, all my respect to him.)* I'm the beast. Like I said, I'm the best.

I'm not as educated as I wish I were, since I took a path through school that was laser-focused on becoming a doctor. I love my career and I take it seriously, but I really wish that instead of taking organic chemistry, I had been able to learn about a wider range of topics. I really wish that my first two years of medical school were not wasted by taking biochemistry all over again. I really wish that I knew more about political science and philosophy and history. I'm lacking so much in history, and I wish I knew more. Teach me some languages. Teach me bass guitar, piano, or art history. What did I accomplish by going to calculus when it has nothing to do with my life? Nothing. Undergraduate education was a complete waste of four years— nothing learned that has helped in my career. I wish I was trained in speaking multiple languages, learning history, political science, philosophy, and more.

Sometimes, I question why I even spent four years in college. Yes, you're supposed to grow up and get away from your parents. You need to make your own bed and clean your own underwear. You're not, however, supposed to take organic chemistry unless you want to be something like the CEO of Schlumberger. If you want to figure out that next place to stick a pipe in the ocean, you might have to take some advanced classes, but they'll be relevant and probably fascinating to you. We should make people learn stuff that they will use in the future. You shouldn't even have a college major. You should be forced to take classes on everything. By focusing on a premed path, I missed out on so much.

That's the reason why, in between building my legacy, I've made it my mission to travel the world. I want to see and learn everything (medical and historic) that I can. I've tried to make up for my lack of a liberal arts education by traveling, and I've been blessed to be able to do so, with private tour guides and archeologists, scientists, and historians to teach me around the world. I've seen medical clinics and pharmacies in many countries. I teach, and I learn. Not only have they afforded me the opportunity to experience a vast range of people and places, cultures and histories, but these travels have also allowed me to observe and even at times to participate within health-care systems around the world.

My travels have taken me from the Andes to Uluru. The best part about Australia was going to Uluru, Ayers Rock. That was the Outback.

I've been to Shanghai, Beijing, Phuket, Hanoi, and Ho Chi Minh City, Cambodia. Dave Weksel and I took our families to see the Terracotta Army in Xi'an. Dave's young daughter Justine, my goddaughter, was a fan: "One time, we went on a trip to China with his whole family," she recalled when "interviewed" for this book. "It was crazy. Like, the weirdest stuff. Cool stuff." (Justine is a bright, precocious child and even goes to Chinese school. "Uncle Steve came along one time," she said. "Afterwards, he played basketball with me in the gym, which was really fun. He wrote some stuff on the whiteboard that made the teacher laugh. And said words in Chinese. Uncle Steve is great.")

In Cambodia, I found the killing fields horrifying. I was fortunate to tour the countryside of Bali, meeting locals and helping them with medical advice. I've been to Tokyo, Mount Fuji, Kyoto. I've been to Delhi, Agra, Jaipur, and Goa, again treating locals. I've swum in the Arabian Sea, the Red Sea, the Dead Sea.

I've been through all parts of Israel from the Red Sea to the Syrian border, and from Jerusalem to the Mediterranean Sea. My desert excursions have included the wonderful sites of Petra, Cairo, the old Nubia, Aswan, and Luxor, not without going to local medical clinics and Hadassah.

I've been to Moscow, St. Petersburg, Estonia, Latvia, Lithuania, Prague. I've been to Odessa, Kiev, Donetsk, and Lugansk, mostly humanitarian trips, but extensive history lessons, nonetheless.

In South America, starting with the Panama Canal, I've been to Buenos Aires and decided to go all the way north to the Argentina-Brazil border at the Iguazu Falls, and south to Patagonia, Ecuador, and the Galapagos Islands. I swam with the turtles and the sea lions and rendered medical advice to locals. My favorite place in South America, though, was my trip to Machu Picchu—this is one for the bucket list.

In South Africa, I took a dip in Shark Alley. I got in the cage, was submerged in water. They throw heads of tunas in the water to attract all the great whites. It worked. There were great whites jumping over the cage with me inside of it. Beyond that, I went to Joberg, and Kruger Park for a safari.

In Europe, I lived in London in the eighties (medical school)—an easy rail ride to Scotland and Wales. Years later, I took my mom, dad, and son all over France, not just Paris. We hit wineries, Champagne places, and the Southern coast.

Germany. My uncle Martin and I drove from Cologne to Dresden into Berlin. I love Prague, but my fav is London. In Spain, Toledo. I don't give a shit about Barcelona. It's just yet another overpopulated and overcrowded cosmopolitan city. If I go to Morocco, I want to go to Gibraltar, Seville, and other parts of Spain on the way. My most memorable European location was in rural northern Greece over Christmas one year, where I treated the entire town of Velvendo. (I was a guest of my dear friend George Klingos.)

On a three-day weekend in Switzerland as medical students, Rob and I went to Interlaken, Montreux, Geneva, and Zurich in one day. That same day, I insisted we take the train into Italy. As it passed through the Northern Italian Alps, we got off the train, got a passport stamp in Domodossola, a northern city in Italy. We exchanged some lire, had pastry, and got back on the train.

The sense of history in Turkey is just indescribable. Visiting Istanbul's Grand Bazaar and standing at the Blue Mosque were very moving experiences.

The former Yugoslavia, including Croatia and the countryside of Dubrovnik and Split, were magnificent. Working my way east, I've rendered medical care in Romania, Copenhagen, Amsterdam, Finland. When in Helsinki, I took that bridge or tunnel to Sweden and turned around and left Sweden.

I've been ten miles from the Sudan border. Great place to see malaria untreated.

I have provided medical care in both Central and Eastern Europe in many countries, and I also have assisted in pharmacies in Southeast Asia, to name a few examples.

I've been virtually all over the US, too. How do I do it while running a booming practice? I take a lot of three- and four-day weekends like that. I love Florence, Rome, and Tuscany, too.

Nothing, however, compares to the journey of fatherhood.

Parents live two lives: we live a life before our children are born, and then we live another life *for* our children, after they are born. I am proud to say that I have a son and a daughter, and being able to see them grow from the size of a melon to grown adults has been gratifying.

There are upsides and downsides, but this is the normal evolutionary life cycle—even for those with money. Some may think that those with money have no problems, but those with money have the same problems as everyone else (except money isn't one of their problems). I don't say this to say I have or don't have money. I use it merely to highlight the fact that rich or poor, we all derive pleasures and knowledge from raising our children. We are all given the gift of children, if we are so lucky, and we should not take our children for granted.

We look to our children for youth, and to teach us how to get older, and how to navigate the Internet. We should use them as a resource, while also sharing our knowledge and encouraging them to scale the peaks of life, to go further than we've ever been. For example, Usain Bolt currently holds the world record at 100 meters. I imagine Bolt would love his son to break his record. He could spend his life imparting the knowledge and training tips that he's learned, and his child might surpass what he accomplished.

I've never had specific career goals picked out for my kids. My only hopes for my children are that they be independent, that they enjoy their own company, and that they enjoy the liberties that I've had, and more. I think we all try to give back to our children more than we were given. It's a natural progression. It's said by many that a billionaire can run out of things to spend money on, but if he or she has children, that's impossible. With kids, there's always something to spend money on.

When it comes to children and money, you don't want them to become too rich too fast, and you don't want them to be drowning in money that they didn't earn, because they won't appreciate it. At the same time, you can get great satisfaction from watching your children dressed up fancy, wearing special costumes or jewelry, driving fancy cars, etc. You can take pleasure and pride from your children going to universities and getting diplomas, traveling to see them graduate. These are all the milestones of life.

My children give me joy and headaches all time. That's a conundrum that they probably won't understand until they are parents themselves. They taught me so much, but above all, they've taught me a lot about responsibility. I used to think that I was a responsible person, until I became a parent. That's sort of like how I tell my friends that I used to think I was in good shape until I started swimming, and then I realized that there was an even higher level of fitness available to me. I call it swim shape.

It's incredible to watch children go through different phases. Mine were very cute and playful at one age, but obnoxious and bratty in others. One of the most exciting parent moments for me was when the kids at less than ten years old would do rounds with me or come to the office: amazing! You must pay your dues as a parent. You must be readily available to change diapers, work, show love and affection, be a good listener, give good advice (whether it's accepted or not!).

No matter what advice I give—whether they're yelling and screaming at me, to me, or for me—even if they appear to hate me at the moment, I know both of my children take my advice to heart. It's such a warm feeling to know that I am responsible for molding their lives. I do believe I am their idol, first love, and best friend, respectively.

What they do with their lives is up to them. My parents always advised me to be self-employed, because they probably knew that I couldn't get along with anybody, or take orders. I want my children to be self-employed as well, so they don't have to take orders from anyone. They deserve to live life with the utmost liberty.

My daughter is a doctor; if she wants to do anything in the medical fields, I am here to help. My father was in the advertising business, and my parents made clear to me was that I should never go into the advertising business. In the same spirit, I've told both of my children that they'll never get wealthy being a doctor. Of course, they won't starve, either. They can certainly be self-employed and make a living in the healthcare field, whether it's nutrition, physical therapy, or a pharmacy—my uncle and maternal grandfather were both pharmacists.

No matter which field they choose, I hope that my children will continue to strive ahead through all the battles, struggles, arguments, torments, and other roadblocks that life has to offer. I hope they will be able to navigate this steeplechase of life with the guidance I have laid down for them. Hopefully, it will make them more successful and less reliant on the system than I ever was.

They are both beautiful people inside and out: loving, caring, warm-hearted. Although they are both extremely intelligent, neither knows as much as they think they do. (That's what I'm here for!) At some point, the tides will turn and they will begin to teach me. I have laid a path for my children to function in society at an outstanding level. Perhaps they will learn all the things that I wish I had learned along the way.

While I didn't learn everything from my parents, all of my desire and will came from them. Watching Dad leave at 6:00 a.m. and return at 7:00

p.m., and Mom would have us wait for father to eat dinner. Dad let Mom run
the home, but she always threatened that Dad would beat my ass when he got
home (if I was out of line). Normal, as I see it. They might not even realize it.
Mom would always talk about nice things, and I knew they were expensive.
I would ask, "Gee, Dad, how come we only go out to Barney's to get me a suit
when it's somebody's bar mitzvah?" The answer *really* was "Because we can't
afford it," but what he said to me was "Well, this is for special occasions."
From that moment on, I wanted my whole life to be a special occasion. I
want that for my children, as well. Mom was always a fixture at Bloomingdales.

To each of them, I have some final thoughts.

Alyx: You're a doctor, you have five years to study and to come into the pro-
verbial family business. With some humility, extra caring, and attentive listening and studying, you will make an outstanding clinician. I will see to it. You
are already an author, a patent holder, and the New York State poster contest
winner for the American College of Physicians. Had it not been for COVID-19,
you would have won in Los Angeles for the national championship.

Jake, my son and the namesake of my grandfather, you are a gentle giant.
Everybody who meets you wants to know which football team was lucky
enough to draft you! And everyone loves your kind, sweet personality. At six
foot one and two hundred and thirty-five pounds, you'll stand on your head
doing push-ups with an eighty-pound vest on until it's dark out. That is a feat
I could never accomplish, and never will. Ultimately, what you do with your
life is more important, though. You are so sweet, kind, loving, and emotional,
and one day you will find the most loving woman to take care of you and give
you children, and keep the Soloway name going. You deserve a wonderful
family that you can watch and raise. You will see your dreams come to frui-
tion once you complete your college degree. I know you will end up becoming
successfully self-employed. Like the rest of us, you have had hurdles in your
working career, but in the end, you will stand at the top of the mountain.

To both of my children, I want to say that you have been a great source of
pride and joy. (I anticipate that this feeling is something that will only continue to grow with age!) The greatest part of being a father is that you are

both individuals, with different needs, wants, and skills. Anything you cannot obtain through me, you will get by following the groundwork I've laid down or through self-discovery. (My parents never heard of a rheumatologist until I became one.)

Even if you don't achieve it, you should always continue searching for the American dream: life, liberty, and the pursuit of happiness. Sometimes one's successes are learned from the ability to cope with failures, all needed life lessons. Unfortunately, in the world we are living in, liberties are sadly more restricted. These are hurdles we will challenge together as a unit. With a little luck from God, though, your own gifts and guidance from me will lead you each to having the perfect life of your own.

The trips that we have taken together have been some of the greatest moments of my life. The more memorable include Auschwitz, China, and Montserrat. Years after the volcano shut down half of the island of Montserrat, I returned with my daughter to the place where I got my start in medicine.

The area where the school once stood is completely engulfed in ash, non-passable to most. The locals, though, were able to tell me when the police weren't going to be in the area, and I was able to hike the volcano with Alyx. (One pleasure, living on the rock, was walking into the live and active volcano, smelling the sulfur, and remembering how soft my skin felt for days after. Many natural springs and waterfalls, quite gorgeous. The other tourist site was a well-hidden plane that lay in wreckage on top of the mountain; sadly, I never saw it.) Under the hot Caribbean sun, we hiked for several miles with a GPS that suddenly stopped functioning. Technically, we were totally off the grid. According to my GPS, we were in the middle of the ocean as we walked above the streets that had been my home during medical school. We hiked for miles and miles and miles before turning back.

All that remains of the school are the lessons that I learned there, the lessons that started me on the path to where I am today. Believe me, I've learned a lot over the years. It's time to share it with the world: the good, the bad, and the ugly. The school did reopen on the Dutch side of the isle of Saint Martin.

CHAPTER 2
HOW HOSPITALS RUINED HEALTHCARE

It is said that we have the best healthcare system in the world, and I suspect that this is largely true. We have the most money, and therefore we tend to have the most accessible and up-to-date treatments. Finding a superb physician can lead to a good outcome much of the time. All of this conceded, however, that does not mean that our system is great. In today's world, medicine has been turned upside down.

Doctors of yesteryear would be rolling in their graves if they could see that the general practitioner or internist no longer sees their own patients when the latter are hospitalized. This is something that started happening fifteen or twenty years ago when some disingenuous people got together and started to create the micromanagement of medicine. Suddenly, hospitals hired physicians (hospitalists) to manage in-patients, thus pushing the general doctor, who cares for these people over the course of a lifetime, out of the picture upon admission. This was all to make the hospital save money, by avoiding too many consultants on the case. Furious house staff feel like secretaries who place orders and spend 95 percent of time typing Medicare compliant notes, but not seeing patients. Sadly, they are robotic and call everyone and leave at 5:00 p.m. sharp. Or the hospitalist may try and take care of the patient far beyond his or her knowledge, and not consult the subspecialists, and the patient's primary care doctor is not involved. If that's true, then you get when you pay for. The sickest patients need a subspecialist and not a doctor they never met before. This is how algorithms and protocols that have destroyed the healthcare system started. Algorithms or protocols are set so the least intelligent will have some clue what to do. The best docs understand protocol and merely use it to teach, or in some cases know better ways to do things. Sadly, adhering only to protocol stifles your ability to think. Nothing can override the experience of a well-trained physician. Similarly, many conditions are diagnosed by criteria. You must understand that criteria are made only to place people in research trials but not diagnose! Again, excellent training and experience will to diagnose lupus, not the criteria! And worse, Medicare only follows protocol! Thinking is prohibited.

There are five specialties: medicine, surgery, pediatrics, obstetrics and gynecology, and psychiatry. Beyond that, there are subspecialties. For example, within the specialty of medicine, one could go on and subspecialize in nephrology, rheumatology, cardiology, gastroenterology, hematology, oncology, and so on. One could do the same in pediatrics: pediatric cardiology, pediatric oncology, pediatric nephrology, etc. So many other specialties and career paths—such as pathology, dermatology, and neurology—do fit into one of the five specialties. However, things changed in recent years.

With the evolving nuances of medicine, which have taken us backward into the Stone Ages, came the invention of what is called a "hospitalist" or "intensivist" if the patient is in the ICU. In the old days, when I trained, we treated the same person in the office, the hospital, or, yes, the ICU. When I trained, we learned those skills. Now, not so much—especially since training hours were cut. Fortunately, some don't follow rules and make trainees stay as long as necessary. Now, they are trained to work shifts, but never to have relationships with patients beyond that. Voilà: the hospitalist was born.

Their work is robotic and instinctive, and they treat everyone the same with little regard for the underlying complexities of an individual patient. Usually, they limit their skills to common situations such as childbirth, gunshot wounds, asthma attacks, heart failure, heart attacks, and gastrointestinal bleeds. They can handily solve the immediate issue, but they never dig deeper. They never stop to learn enough about the patient to find out what was the cause of that incident. Even more pressingly, they never ask, "What is the appropriate long-term follow-up and treatment?"

So, from family doctors who would stay with patients for generations, our system has evolved backward to shift workers who might treat you for five minutes. That wasn't the worst of it, though. Then came the onslaught of international medical grads, physician extenders, and additional medical students, some osteopath and some allopath. The government pays hospitals for training spots. The hospitals use that money to buy practices. It's easier for the government to keep an eye on fewer hospitals than more doctors.

(For those of you who don't think discrimination and racism exist in our hospitals, think again. If you are an international medical grad, and you think you can have the same choices as a US citizen that went to a US medical school, you've got another thing coming. You either have to rely on nepotism or massive donations to gain a prestigious spot if you are not a home-grown doctor. These words cannot be echoed loud enough.)

Sadly, for today's patients, a hospital admission is no longer just a tumultuous trial by fire; it is a disaster. They are greeted by nurses who are fresh out of school and slaves to protocol, which unfortunately always panders to the lowest common denominator. Some seem to avoid the use of critical thinking—perhaps due to lack of training, perhaps due to an egomaniac sociopath at the helm of their hospital. Either way, deviation from the rulebook is not allowed, no matter how it may benefit the patient.

You are not allowed to get an IV started with your arm numb anymore, for example. You just have to suffer with the big needle, and you have to hope that the nurse or phlebotomist who comes to your room knows how to do it on the first try. Why? I've been told that fifteen years ago at one major institution, there was a shortage of Novocain. When they found that the IV insertion worked out OK without using it, they decided to save money and never reordered it for that purpose again. That hospital saved a few dollars, and every patient since who's gotten an IV has suffered in pain. It's very sad. This clearly shows that the system will always look for ways to save money rather than to do what is just right. In fact, if the patient is numb, it is much easier for the person starting the IV because the patient will not jump around and move. The new way may cost more, since more needles end up being wasted when the patient is in pain and can't sit still. That means that the patient does not have to be stuck more than once, which risks damaging their vein, causing many potential complications such as phlebitis. That's just where the bad care begins.

Say you wake up in the morning in your hospital bed; you ask for your doctor, and you are told a doctor will see you soon. If need be, you'll get IV water to prolong your stay so they generate hospital revenue. Then, a group comes into your room—spearheaded by someone you've never seen before, who is obviously in a rush. These people are often employed by the hospital, or perhaps they are employed by a group of physicians. Their only goal is to see the patient as fast as possible and get out of the hospital. All the while, the patient and families are—justifiably—asking, "Where is the doctor?" Before long they'll find out the brutal truth: doctors just don't go to hospitals anymore.

It is unfortunate, but there is no more continuity of care. In years past, if a doctor fell off the planet, his or her patients would have cried in harmony. Now, everybody would rush to the Internet and find a new doctor as fast as possible. In many cases, the only information they would use to make their decision would be computer programs, Yelp reviews, and insurance company recommendations.

This all creates a colossal waste of money. In the era of rising drug costs, we are brainwashed from TV and newspapers to believe that medical costs are out of control because pharmaceutical companies are ripping off the public. That is just not entirely true (the rip-off is the golden parachute and yearly new CEO). Let me explain why with an example.

Rheumatoid arthritis often overlaps with Hepatitis C. So, I personally diagnosed and referred one thousand patients to my local gastroenterologist for Hepatitis C treatment. At that time, the treatment included alpha interferon. Many of the patients were never cured. In addition, many experienced liver failure, liver cancer, liver transplants, and other serious scenarios. Those additional scenarios ended up costing more than one million dollars per patient for hospital admission and full treatment protocol. Meanwhile, the medicine that would have cured the problem to begin with was eighty thousand dollars. Eighty thousand dollars times all the people who were afflicted by a terrible life-threatening disease is a huge cost. It would have been all but eradicated if the insurance company had let them get the eighty-thousand-dollar drug, which was actually a bargain at the time. In fact, this one drug ultimately was so successful, the pharmaceutical company is running out of patients and is no longer as strong a company as it once was. The happy ending here: people get the drug, and hepatitis C is no longer a condition filling hospital with liver failures and liver transplants that cost millions.

Other examples of waste that are becoming ubiquitous in medicine include the treatment of inflammatory disease such as rheumatoid arthritis, psoriatic arthritis, the arthritis of inflammatory bowel disease (ulcerative colitis and Crohn's), or sarcoid arthritis, just to name a few. These conditions are treated with medications that cost somewhere in the neighborhood of two thousand dollars a month. Again, people wail and moan about the price, blaming Big Pharma. The patients are told that the price of the drug is inflated by the need to administer the drug in a hospital. That is totally outrageous. Fortunately, these drugs given in the doctor's office are very cost-effective and keep arthritics out of hospitals. (Now that Big Pharma doesn't wine or dine docs anymore, where did that billion go?)

I have lobbied politicians for twenty years to ask that these drugs be administered in doctors' offices. This would make the price anywhere from 60 to 90 percent cheaper than the administration in a hospital. Why? There is no hospital fee. There is no charge for a Tylenol or a Band-Aid. At a doctor's office, all that is included. In the hospital, it could cost forty bucks just to open the Band-Aid, and an extra forty to put it on. There is no reason for outpatients to be practically bankrupted when being treated. (Have your infusion medicine in a doctor's office only.)

My practice model includes on-site administration of biologic drugs. Why is this important, beyond the savings to patients? 1. There is 100 percent success with compliance, and 2. To repeat, the injectable drugs in the office are cheaper than the self-injectable drugs, as long as they are given in the office, not the hospital.

However, some of the more pompous Ivy League doctors think they are going to save the world from spending extra money and refuse to offer their patients the intravenous drugs. Intravenous drugs have more direct and better absorption, but if you are a patient at one of the Harvard University teaching hospitals, your last choice will be the IV drug Infliximab. Instead, they will give you the subcutaneous injection Humira. (By no means is it a better drug. It only suits the needs of the institution and punishes the patient, who is clueless to this, as there is no place *they* will infuse their patients.) The holier-than-thou doctors (usually leftists) don't think about which drug might be best for the patient in the long term. Instead, they make the executive decision that those IV drugs are simply too expensive to use. You would think they were the ones paying for it.

In fact, these academic doctors are getting *paid* for it. They get hundreds of thousands of dollars or even millions of dollars from pharmaceutical companies as stock options, dividends, and other creative means of payment. No one's true salary is ever really known because of all these kickbacks. Everybody who is in the top one-tenth of a percent seems to have the same low salary, but they have a lot of other slush to pad it out.

With shady business going on behind the scenes, how can you pick a doctor who will have your best interests at heart? Sadly, most people feel that all doctors are the same. When choosing a doctor, they look for convenience: the closest doctor with the shortest waiting time for an appointment. Unfortunately, this is the exact *opposite* of what you should do. Every doctor is different. The quality of each doctor is different. The diagnostic abilities of every doctor who different. Our training is different. While the anatomy and the information may be the same, that is where it ends. Sadly, many patients suffer by taking the easy way out.

Should you look for certain degrees, or fancy alma maters? It is not necessary to have trained at an Ivy League institution. I'm not saying that to cover up the fact that I did not go to an Ivy League institution; it's the truth. As I preach to anyone who will listen, patients should not shop any institution, but rather, look for the reputation of an excellent physician or clinician.

Some of the best doctors I know are from Ivy League institutions. However, some of the worst are, as well. Overall, there are more bad than good doctors, and people should keep that in mind. It is unfortunate, as I believe most people are well intended. It goes back to the fact that the new wave of doctors looks at medicine as a shift-work position and nothing more.

I had a stunning experience recently that drove home the harsh reality of the rise of the hospitalist. I was speaking on the telephone with a hospital-based physician regarding one of my patients, when they interrupted me at 5:10 p.m. to tell me that the call had to end. Why? They said, "It is no longer work time. It's mommy time." I asked, "Are you a shift worker?" and the doctor replied, "Yes, I am a shift worker. You will have to speak with one of my associates." This wasn't much help, since her associates were also shift workers, and they had never seen or heard of the patient whom we were discussing at that point.

If you're not getting it by now, this system is terrible for patient care, and it must change. There must be absolute continuity of care, with the primary physician seeing their own patients in the hospital. Hospitalists should be what moonlighters used to be: extra help at night in case there are true emergencies that need to be dealt with. Of course, they shouldn't be awakened every five to ten minutes to see if somebody can take an over-the-counter medicine. This should be the responsibility of the nurse caring for the patients. As I have seen, however, the shift-work attitude has affected nursing, too. No one seems to know what is wrong with the patient at any given time, and without the order of the physician, nurses are often banned from doing something as simple as giving a patient ice chips or hard candy.

Pre-op patients are NPO (nothing by mouth), after midnight. While a nurse following protocol would be told by the doctor that the principle is that food in the stomach may end up in the lungs when surgery and or anesthesia occurs, an intelligent caregiver will learn and understand a sip of water at 1:00 a.m. is safe. The old days of thoughtful nursing would dictate the experienced nurses knew that within eight hours or less a patient can have a lozenge, not a hoagie! The new nurses of today read the protocol and don't ask what the exceptions may be to comfort someone. If the patient had trouble with extubation, often morbidly obese with many comorbidities, they could aspirate (when food from your stomach ends up in your lungs). However, these people should use their heads. (In fact, there should be protocols for healthy vs. unhealthy patients.) Aspiration would never be an issue if someone ate an ice chip or licked a hard candy, or had a sip of water twelve hours ago. You would not be adding much more to their normal gastric secretions. I myself have had a hard candy in my mouth on the way to the operating room. I just spit it out when I got there.

The rules exist for a reason, but they are never balanced out with common sense. They're followed too strictly because we must always cater to the lowest common denominator—or perhaps the person who didn't belong in the profession in the first place just doesn't care.

Yes, believe it or not, there are people in medicine who just show up for the paycheck and don't care at all. They don't want to work. They *do* want to be looked at in high esteem. They want to be treated—and paid—better than the average person. They want to be recognized for their extra education. They want to be recognized and patted on the back for all the lives they allegedly saved and all the people they allegedly helped. This is why so many physicians go to larger health systems, where they can get a check for sub-par work.

Of course, there are highly motivated professionals in all types of medicine. They include the physician's assistants, nurse practitioners, registered nurses, physicians, and even students who work pushing wheelchairs. It does not matter at which level a physician is in their career. They all have the ability to show concern and care for the patient. It does not take a lot of effort to do, and being aware of your patients is often the difference between life and death. Certainly, in the aging population, the comfort of seeing a familiar face or a consistent face is extremely important. It helps to fend off depression and irritability in addition to the medical problem that brought them in for medical care in the first place.

How can we train people to follow their brains and hearts instead of the rulebook and the clock? Today's training is somewhere between bad and awful. With the training hours being cut, the most important time to learn is when you're on your own at night, so you can then discuss the answers with the attending physician in the morning. (If you're a first-year resident, you're hoping to learn from someone with more experience!) However, these opportunities rarely occur.

Today's system is geared toward teaching less and pushing out more people. No one is able to get enough practical experience because of work-hour limitations. Big government and big business have forced this form of socialized medicine on us. People always say, "My doctor didn't spend five minutes with me." If the doctor is motivated to make money, he can't spend more than five minutes with you. (They look at computer screens, not you!) I don't agree with having shorter hours for training, and I don't agree with doctors working a nine-to-five schedule, either.

In a nine-to-five job, employed by a system and not yourself, people don't care nearly as much. If you haven't married YOUR business, your business will fail! The VA is a perfect example of failure of care and wasting unlimited money.

It's disgraceful that the system no longer has family doctors seeing all the patients at the hospital at all times. Instead, we have doctors who barely speak English, which makes it difficult for them to connect with some patients. It intimidates the elderly. Most just rummage around saying hello to all the patients, hoping they can improve by osmosis so they can go home before the insurance denies their admissions. Patient care would be better if all the doctors spoke a very high level of English, so people would not have to struggle to understand them on top of everything else.

However, not all hospitals are alike. In fact, there are crucial differences between what I would call a "university" hospital and a "community" hospital. In theory, the "brightest" doctors—a.k.a. those with a high GPA—are at the university hospital, while the highly motivated ones who were B and C students are at the community hospital. Those at community hospitals tend to do a lot of work, because the patients tend to be underinsured, perhaps with Medicaid, and often don't have good advocates. Anybody with a white coat is good enough to be a doctor, according to the patient or the family in these particular hospital settings.

At the university hospital, on the other hand, you allegedly have all of your straight-A students, and the system is very sterile. There is often little participation or hands-on work done by the trainees. When they are ready to start their own careers, they have virtually no real experience.

On the flip side, at the community hospital the trainees do everything. They learn how to speak to sick patients and how to recognize various crises much better than those trained in the university setting. However, they lack the connections to the renowned researchers and often don't get their names in the bright lights.

A third option—probably the worst option—is the urgent care centers. Like hospitals, urgent care centers come in two general types. The first category consists of those owned by hospitals. They typically charge from $100 to $200 to let you walk in the door, only to send you to the hospital, where your insurance will get charged another few thousand dollars. (By the way, you are not credited back your original fee from the urgent care, and that is double-dipping on the part of the hospital.)

The second type of urgent care center is the kind owned by a group of physicians. It is truly amazing how a patient can call their doctor for an emergency and be told, "I'm sorry, we're busy today. Try the urgent care center down the street." They don't tell the patient that the doctor is the one who's going to benefit. Meanwhile, that fifty- to seventy-five-dollar office visit just became a one-hundred- to two-hundred-dollar urgent care visit. Systems like this incentivize doctors to take time off and attract doctors who are somewhat disinterested to begin with. This is the truth, and this is how medicine works.

Overall, I would say that pretty much everything that the general public thinks they know about the medical system is untrue, especially when it comes to hospital care. Is there any way to make the system better, and to ensure a continuum of care when hospitalists and shift workers run rampant? I would challenge the health workers out there who really care to break away from the lowest common denominator. That means deviating from protocol and actually using your brain.

Protocols tend to be the standard of care, and breaking them allows attorneys to sue physicians or medical boards to crucify them. Still, the smartest and most experienced physicians never follow protocol because they are too good at what they do, which leads to fights and audits with insurance carriers. A protocol exists so that the lowest common denominator on the totem pole has some clue what to do in case an issue comes up. With that fact in mind, it is truly sad that there needs to be any protocols at all. It shows the lack of knowledge and the acceptance of ignorance in what should be a very well-qualified system.

One example of "protocol" is having a major hospital system to begin with. Another might be having an as-needed order for the use of Narcan on all postoperative hospital patients. The dreadful psychological trauma induced by receiving Narcan may be great for a heroin addict, but it has no place in mainstream society and should never be administered to a normal patient. The use of Narcan, then, is one example where patient evaluation should win out over protocol.

Other needed deviations from protocol come at a political level. When someone graduates medical school, they go on to postgraduate training. Your first year is referred to as your internship, which is part of your residency. The state that you're doing it in requires you to have a training license. Depending on the state you're practicing in, you can get your unrestricted license in your second year—meaning you can work as a physician on your own even without finishing your training. Once you've finished training and you go into practice, there is then the opportunity to become board-certified. Before you're board-certified, you are called board-eligible, and you remain that way for eight years. If you lose your board-eligibility, you're not allowed to take the board certification exam unless you do repeated training. The scary thing is that to get a license, you only have to go to the training. You don't have to get certified.

Interestingly, most hospitals within a state will not allow you on the staff unless you are board-certified. (Doesn't matter; those docs don't go anyway.) There seems to be a paradox here that I don't understand. Why do we have a certification exam if one does not need to be able to pass the exam in order to be a practicing doctor?

Furthermore, half the lawmakers seem to have no idea that this is a statute of regulations. When trying to prosecute physicians in the state, they continually ask each defendant of any infraction, "Are you board-certified?" The answer should be, "Why do you care? It doesn't matter in this state."

It's not just the protocol. We have too many outdated laws in our society. One example is in the state of Virginia. Did you know that if you are a pedestrian and get run over by a car in Virginia, you're the one at fault? I guess you shouldn't have been jaywalking when that car was coming. For some reason or another, that law has never been updated to meet the realities of modern society.

In the same way, the doctor-patient relationship has changed drastically, and the old rulebook needs to be thrown out. The patients do not see their own physicians when they go to a hospital, which is when they need their physician the most. Instead, they're seen by a hospitalist who swears by protocol. Unfortunately, protocol has changed, and patients suffer for it. Twenty years ago, there was better training with more hands-on supervision. There were more bedside rounds, more meetings, and more conferences. So many of these things no longer occur. Perhaps that means doctors have more free time, but it hasn't improved patient care. Instead, all of these changes have resulted in fewer smart people going into medicine. They want nothing to do with the modern hospitals that have made medicine into a mill and a factory, rather than a healthcare facility.

Clearly, the hospitalists have not made the system better. I've seen the brutal results of these changes firsthand.

CHAPTER 3
BAD MEDICINE

One day, I saw this guy—a total sad sack—limping around my apartment building in Manhattan. I said, "What the hell is wrong with you?!"

He said, "You probably haven't heard of this, but I have gout. I'm from Australia, and I have to fly back soon, but I'm in too much pain for a long flight."

"Well, it just so happens that I'm the best gout doctor in the country. Get yourself to my office. It's a hundred miles south of here. I'll see you when you get there."

He said, "Well, I'm leaving in two days. Can I come tonight or tomorrow?"

I said, "Come first thing tomorrow morning. You don't have to pay; you don't have to sign in; you don't have to do anything."

The next day, he got a limo to take him down to Jersey. I took off his shoes and socks, identified inflamed joints and tendons, took some fluid, confirmed it was gout, injected joints and tendons. He got up off the table and he said, "They would never do this in Australia!"

I said, "They wouldn't do this in Manhattan, either. That's why I'm the best." He is still a patient and ten years of no gout attacks and well controlled under my guidance.

Like I said, you can go to the biggest, fanciest, most prestigious hospital there is, but that doesn't mean you'll see a good doctor, let alone a top one-percent doctor. (Oh, by the way, the top lists are crap, too. Remember, it's all whom you may know, or who may want you kept off a list. There is no court of appeals for this.)

There are many idiots there, too. In fact, you often see a neophyte who knows nothing, hence don't get sick in July when the new residents start.

Many idiots have gray hair, too. I'll explain. I arrived in 1993, got on staff, etc. I had to submit my first ten cases for review, I was assigned a preceptor. Sadly, he didn't know what a rheumatologist was!

Just when you thought this story was done, I was called to a consultation and was promptly followed into the patient's room by a curmudgeon. (A gentleman who was unkempt and looked out of place but was my senior at the hospital in his field.) He watched with bated breath as I did my history and physical exam and made conclusions. He asked, "What are your thoughts?" I replied that the patient has lymphoma. He smirked and asked, "How do you know that?" to which I answered, "You just watched everything I did. What more can I explain? That's my conclusion." Short story (LYMPHOMA+). This was our first encounter.

Our next meeting occurred in a public hallway at a different hospital. He announced, "You killed so and so." My reply: "If you have nothing intelligent to say, then go fuck yourself and stay away from me." In spite of my world-class reputation, he forced people who needed my care to avoid me. He made a career of it. In a clandestine manner, his associates sent patients for my quality of care.

The icing on the cake is when the woman (mentioned in this book) who spent ten days dying was diagnosed by me in five minutes—this got his goat. Although always a curmudgeon, he became a dotard! The guy is jealous as the day is long. He has conned the other docs a lot but was unopposed until I arrived. I heard from a hospitalist that enjoys my great work; he told me I found an infection that was missed by the doctor. This person routinely puts fear in patients rather than comforting them.

Doctors are just like baseball players. They go where they get the best contract, not where the patient care is good. It's sad that they're not self-employed, so they're not motivated. Lives are lost, lives are ruined because of this.

I had a patient with Class IV lupus nephritis admitted to the hospital. It took me five days and two hours of phone calls every night to finally get the patient to receive the medicine she needed. This patient, who needed life-or-death treatment for kidney failure related to lupus, was delayed five days because of technical bullshit.

Nobody at the hospital wanted to do their job. They all just passed the buck, shift to shift. I wrote the orders myself on Tuesday night, and the excuses began.

"There's no nurse in the hospital able to give a chemo-type drug."

"We don't carry that drug."

"The pharmacist won't give that drug," because they don't understand the package inserts. Often medications are used off-label, achieving great effect. (A package insert only lists the approved uses by FDA, as determined by which conditions the pharma company applied for, and nothing more—that's the sad truth, you have to apply for that indication, and it's a long process.)

Suffice to say, the person who was supposed to take care of it didn't. I called up to see if the patient tolerated the drug. They didn't even know what I was talking about. I gave a verbal order to the nurse, and she said, "No problem. We'll take care of it."

I called the next day and asked, "How did the patient do?" They claimed there were no orders for the drug they were supposed to administer the night before. I then found out that this drug I'm ordering isn't even in the system at the hospital! So I had a near donnybrook with the head of the pharmacy, and they agreed to prepare the drug and give it to the patient the following morning. They had to fax me a consent form, which I signed and sent back. As far as I was concerned, we were good to go.

Meanwhile, the poor guy's daughter was calling all day asking what was going on, and I said, "I took care of all the paperwork, and I'll be by tonight after work to see how it all went." When I showed up, there was a nurse sitting there on the stool in the room, and I'm like, "Hey, who are you?"

She said she was the chemo nurse, which didn't help me understand the situation any better. I said, "Uh, why are you here?"

She goes, "Well, I'm required to be here when we're giving Cytoxan."

And I said, "Why? We give this in my office on a regular basis."

She goes, "Well, this isn't your office."

I took a deep breath and counted to ten before I said, "Listen, why are you here so late, though? I got the paperwork signed, sealed, delivered by 10:30 a.m."

She says, "Well this is when I got here. I started at 4:00 p.m."

Yes, the patient eventually got the drug he needed from the hospital. Because it took five days, though, he's currently on dialysis and suffered permanent damage.

Another night, I had a pharmacist refuse to give a drug to a patient with kidney failure from lupus. They called me at one o'clock in the morning to tell me that. I said, "I can tell you from looking at him that that's the only treatment that will work. Otherwise he will die!"

This person said to me, "Well, I was reading the package insert, and it says you can't give it to kidney failure." That's true if you're a breast cancer patient, but we were dealing with lupus. Lupus is immune-mediated. I said, "This is going to kill the antibodies. That's the only drug that works." Long story short, the patient ended up getting it at seven or eight o'clock in the morning. He stopped screaming because he was all good. I was yelling, "I'm a board-certified rheumatologist. This is what I do for a living!"

All of that red tape and blind allegiance to protocol hurts the patients in the end. Another example of that is one of my patients who had aortitis, an inflammation of the aorta. The aorta is a large blood vessel that carries oxygen from the heart. So, the patient was short of breath, and since you shouldn't be short of breath unless you have aortic heart valve disease, we had to look for other options.

To get to the heart of the problem (pun intended), we'd have to get what's called a right heart catheterization, which measures the pressure within the lungs. Well, the insurance company denied that, and the patient never got the test. (They often deny testing and force patients to delayed diagnosis.) The insurance company *did* keep allowing echocardiograms, which give an **estimate** of the lung pressure. Every day, the patient got another echocardiogram, and we never got any closer to having a solid idea of how the lungs were working. We wasted $500 a day in echocardiograms instead of just getting the patient a cath in the beginning for $1,000.

To this day, that patient *still* hasn't got the cath, and they *still* don't really know what's going on. If we could determine that the patient truly has pulmonary hypertension (the cause of shortness of breath we are searching for), we have three classes of drugs that we could use to treat it. However, if aortitis is the cause of the shortness of breath, and we can prove that by ruling out everything else, then we are in a canoe in a river and we at least know where we're headed. Our paddle would be small, but at least we'd have one. Now, because of the insurance company, that patient is totally rudderless.

Just the other day was a horror story that illustrates how these small, seemingly random decisions can change someone's whole life. I was treating a woman suffering from health problems for years and was incorrectly diagnosed. The woman in her history was known to have had fourteen miscarriages—each time within the first month of gestation. Nobody ever checked to see if she had a lupus anticoagulant blood test. I found it odd, and I did in fact discover that her lupus anticoagulant was present on more than one occasion. Therefore, had this woman taken an anticoagulant, she would never have lost her babies. Too bad it was too late for her to have kids by the time we figured it out. Her mistreatment was just heartbreaking.

In another case, I recall a lady referred to me for a positive rheumatoid factor years ago. With rheumatoid factor positive, it may not be rheumatoid arthritis, lupus, or a couple of other things. It could be a monoclonal immunoglobulin deposition disease, for example.

The patient comes down, I look through a couple of the papers and say, "Your rheumatoid factor's positive. Do you have any joint pain?"

She says, "Nope. No pain at all."

I'm like, "Let me ask you something. If you have no pain, why did your doctor test you for rheumatoid factors and send you to me?"

She said, "Oh I think it was routine testing," but it's not part of any routine testing, and it shouldn't be. (An example of "pretest probability.")

I started looking more through her papers and said, "Well, tell me more about your background," and she tells me she had breast cancer, which was diagnosed about five years ago. I ask her, "What kind of breast cancer did you have?" and she gives me this blank stare. I was like, "You don't know."

She says, "Well, I never did the breast biopsy."

Wow. If you never got a breast biopsy, how do you know if you had breast cancer?! She claimed, "It was my lymph node. I never had breast tissue biopsied."

My brain started spinning. I just wanted to kill somebody for giving her that kind of treatment. And, I have a suspicion. I ask her, "Do you have dry eyes and dry mouth?" She told me she has severe dryness—of the eyes and mouth. With the positive rheumatoid factor, and further a lip biopsy, she met the diagnostic criteria for Sjogren's Syndrome. The dummy who diagnosed breast cancer without a breast biopsy actually didn't know that the patient had lymphoma related to Sjogren's and never had breast cancer in the first place. Sjogren's is usually treatable if you catch it soon enough, but in the end, that patient died. What a travesty. (Speaking of Sjogren's, Venus Williams, please call me if you want to manage your Sjogren's better on and off the court.)

I was very new to the area. I had only been in practice for about two or three days. There was a buzz in the air. Everybody knew that a rheumatologist had arrived. A patient apparently had severe abdominal pain, with a diagnosis of lupus and no rheumatologist. The patient did not get treated properly. In fact, anything but. My phone rings from a surgeon (who was likely drunk) calling from the operating room. (By the way, drunk physicians operating is not something I have not seen before. Nor have I shied away from noticing that nurses and doctors alike have rushed from sex in the call room to the operating room. You want to make sure that your surgeon is happy before he gets to the work that day. I've also seen nurses punching doctors, doctors punching students, and people throwing metal objects at others—a specific recollection was a neurosurgeon punching a student in the chest while both were over the open spine, the student falling backward.)

The surgeon indicated that he had a patient with lupus and very severe pain on the operating table. The pain was so severe, he said, that he had to cut the patient open. Little did he know that proper medication would have resolved everything almost immediately, as is the case in nearly all abdominal pain in lupus patients. The spleen was the largest he had ever seen in his life, and he wanted to know what to do next, since he removed it. My advice was to put the spleen back immediately or the patient would likely die from having so much of their blood removed. A spleen that big could be holding two or more liters of the patient's blood. In fact, the patient died unnecessarily within twenty to thirty minutes of the phone call.

In the same vein, about 15 years ago, lupus patients, as they still do, constantly get admitted to the hospital with pericardial disease, which means fluid around the heart. The proper treatment is to administer intravenous steroids; however, unless I'm called, unneeded surgery called pericardial window or pericardial stripping is performed. This is completely unnecessary 99.9 percent of the time. I had a stern conversation with the thoracic surgeon and told him to never do this procedure again on an autoimmune patient without calling me first. And for ten years, until that doctor moved to Florida, we never had another surgery for a pericardial window on a lupus patient in our health system.

I'm not making these up. These are the real-life consequences of a broken system. I could go on with bad medicine stories longer than I have in my life to write about!

I don't think anything is more appalling than having a patient seen with a hot, swollen, tender, red foot, who can't bear weight on it, and being told without an X-ray that they have a broken foot or ankle. They're in a cast, which only makes the real problem—a gout attack—even worse. These people have to go home and saw the cast off themselves, they're in so much pain. Not only have I seen it once, but I've seen it twice, thrice, and then some.

This is why when a patient finds me, they know they've found the best. Just this week, I had a patient drive six hours to my office from Boston. Apparently, nobody in Boston was able to diagnose, treat, and control his gout fast enough for his wife. He will not go anywhere else. He doesn't care if he pays cash or not, and personally I don't even know what insurance he has. I believe he is of Medicare age. This is a man who has access to plenty of care in Boston but needs to drive six hours for *proper* care.

I'm not nitpicking at my colleagues; frankly they can't do things the way I do. I have a patient, Christopher Lotz, who drives regularly from New Orleans, Louisiana, with a spondyloarthropathy. He found me on YouTube and says I'm the only doctor he ever found who can actually explain things in a straightforward, cohesive manner.

I performed a history, physical, and X-rays and came to a pretty conclusive decision that he has spondyloarthropathy. I told him he needed treatment with a biologic agent. He'd finally found relief, because he'd found the best. Months later, though, he called and said it's too far for him to keep driving back and forth from New Orleans. I told him, "Take my records and my notes. Go to New Orleans and find a rheumatologist. Give them my notes and just tell them you want to continue your care there."

After taking my notes back to New Orleans and sharing my notes with four rheumatologists in New Orleans, he found that they agreed with everything I said. Perfect, right? The only problem was, they decided they wouldn't follow my directions after they Googled me and found out that I graduated from medical school in a foreign country. They all told him that my information couldn't be trusted. Ironically, he asked, "Well, if you don't believe Soloway, can you tell me what I *do* have?" Nobody had an answer. "Why did Dr. Soloway's treatment plan work?" Again, no answer. This is an example of a tragic ego issue by a feckless doctor.

He explained that I give him Infliximab, and methotrexate for a spondyloarthropathy. They didn't believe it would work. Now, even though he would prefer to get his treatment at home in Louisiana, he still comes 1,350 miles several times a year and sleeps in a mobile home park because I am the only one who has ever been able to give him relief. Just recently, he was able to find a physician specializing in pain management who agreed with me on all counts and is helping to coordinate care for the patient in his hometown. I am elated he is such a nice man.

One of my patients will fly in just for the day from Tampa. He does not trust or allow anybody to inject his knee other than me.

Apparently, doctors who have been trained within the past twelve to fifteen years have either been going to bed early, waking up late, or following government guidelines that limit the hours they can learn in the hospital system. Whether this is the reason or not, the quality of care is going downhill—not staying the same and not getting better. Unless your title is president of the United States, you wait in long lines and hope to get mediocre care, even though you and everyone else think their doctor is the best. Frankly, I do not think the physicians taking care of the president are all that good, either. (A generalization—not referring to anyone in particular.) In fact, prior to his winning the election in 2016, we sat down to discuss a condition that afflicted someone he knows. When I was done explaining, his comment was, "Why is there no one in my home city, other than you? You are the only one who can explain this topic and I understand what you are talking about!" Your doctor friends aren't the best. I am. Nearly every patient I've ever had would agree. This excludes the ones that I couldn't help, because their issues were in another field. There was nothing I could do; still, they hate me even if I refer them to a great doctor who can help.

You sit in my office and complain about the multihour wait. You can't comprehend that I know what's wrong and how to fix it in five minutes. You're mad because I didn't hold your hand, and you forget how many wasted visits and copays you had with all the reckless or feckless doctors, and simply those who have no idea what a good rheumatologist—or the best rheumatologist, in my case—can do for you. They say you need a great accountant and lawyer; I say you need a great rheumatologist.

I lose my temper and I get very angry sometimes at the other doctors, and I tell people, "You've been trusting your family doctor for ten years, and your family doctor has referred you to physical therapy, a chiropractor, an acupuncturist, an orthopedic surgeon, a neurosurgeon, maybe even a different rheumatologist. I'm sitting here a mile from that person's office. They either don't know who I am, or they would rather send you to their friends than to me, as they don't want you to come here. It's probably the latter, because I've been in practice twenty-eight years. That's sad because they're taking out their feelings of jealousy about me on you.

They know the best care is here. They don't have your best interest at heart, and that's when it's time for you to get a new doctor."

Even I can be stymied by the quagmire that is Big Pharma, however. The biggest factor in this mess is the testing system, which is always evolving and changing. I'm not certain what the right answer is, as to which test and which format would best identify useful new drugs. However, I do understand that if a system is continually changing for no particular reason, it means that whoever makes up the testing has no idea what is going on.

If there is no perfect treatment, there are usually ten adequate treatments. If ten people have rheumatoid arthritis and all ten are on a different biologic drug, this is simply because nobody has shown that one drug is a lot better than the other drugs. There are reasons why one drug would be preferred from one doctor to the next. Perhaps it's because of the method of administration: if a drug can be given through an IV, it will be absorbed better than injecting it, and much better than going through a stomach. (Stomachs more than fifty years old also have an especially poor absorption ability.) What doesn't make sense is why—if there are ten drugs that are all considered to be adequate—a drug company is allowed to continue producing similar drugs. This is a total waste of energy, effort, and money, when novel treatments could be developed instead. It's utterly ludicrous that there are more than thirty NSAIDs (like Aspirin, Motril, and Advil) available and that people actually prescribe them.

A thought: until we have treatment for brain cancer and Alzheimer's, we should have no more arthritis drug development. No more "me toos"!

The paucity of drugs for some diagnoses—and the lack of appropriate testing on those that *do* exist—makes treating patients with the best care next to impossible at times. This happens, for example, when there is no medication indicated.

Once, I had a patient with large vessel vasculitis who needed a drug called Rituximab. However, the Rituximab routinely gets denied, because it's not indicated. You might say to me, "Steve, why would you give something not indicated? Why don't you use what is indicated?" (A drug can be the standard of care yet not be indicated merely because the pharmaceutical company didn't fill out the paperwork. But the better doctors know and inherently fight for their patients.) Many diseases have virtually nothing indicated, so should we send all people home and assume the canard?

I'd say, "That's a good question! There haven't been enough trials, and therefore, nothing is indicated." We do what we're supposed to do. We do what works, and we make the patients better. There's nothing indicated for large vessel vasculitis officially, but you have to use what works. Now, we usually start with prednisone—steroids—and that's great. Once they respond, you can convert them to Rituximab, which we know works. Depending on the type of vasculitis, sometimes we have even better options than that. Still, they're not approving anything.

Before I even prescribe a patient a biologic drug, the first thing I do is check what kind of insurance they have. You are often forced to use what the insurance company prefers. Insurance companies prefer some drugs over others because of side deals they cut with the manufacturers. If, for example, they buy a cancer drug from Company X, Company X will give them rebates or will lower their price—provided the insurance company promises all the business for Drug Z. We should obviously be able to use the most appropriate drug for the patients. There are nuances—especially with increasing experience—that would allow one to choose a more appropriate treatment for individual patients.

That means the best doctors have to look beyond the law of "protocol" if they want to keep patient care and comfort front and center.

Guidelines are like speed limits, and you really need to understand the background to know that if the speed limit is sixty-five and it's snowing, you're going to drive thirty, and on a sunny day on the Jersey Turnpike, you're going to go eighty. Guidelines are written for research protocols, and they do not always fit with proper treatment of a patient. I'm not going to say that they're completely wrong, but there are much better ways than what is portrayed in many guidelines. Anyone with enough experience can make their own guidelines. Academic doctors are forced to make guidelines that make no sense so they can get patients for their research trials and keep their jobs.

The same goes for being board-certified. Being board-certified doesn't mean you're good. It means you know the minimum to proceed with work. I was reminded of this fact by a former friend and colleague, Antonio Reginato, who is deceased. He was a true leader in both academics and clinical care.

Take lupus of the kidneys, lupus nephritis. There's a kazillion people with lupus, like three percent of the population, but there's no cure for it. We all prescribe cyclophosphamide monthly for six months. How can we use it when there's no treatment approved? It's cheap, so nobody cares.

And then there's Cellcept, a drug indicated for transplant rejection. It's currently the standard of care for a subset of lupus patients, but Genentech Pharmaceutical never applied for the lupus indication. Since they never applied, it's not indicated for lupus, yet it's the standard of care for lupus nephritis. (It just so happens that there's a drug that will be released in the next six-to-twelve months that will be mixed with Cellcept, and it may take over as the new protocol. The trials look good.)

If you do all these things and go the extra mile to actually put your patients first, you'll have a patient for life. This kind of doctor-patient relationship is becoming increasingly rare.

One of my patients had been going to the hospital almost every weekend—as a young man!—because his doctors were getting his diagnosis all wrong. For five years prior to meeting me, he would tell his doctors that he didn't feel well. They would check his sed rate and C-reactive protein, which are markers of inflammation, and if they were too high, he would be inappropriately admitted to the hospital for the weekend for no reason. (We do not treat blood tests; we treat the patient's symptoms.) Sometimes he'd feel totally fine and end up in the hospital. Other times, he actually *did* feel sick, but they did nothing because the test was "normal." This went on and on and on until I met him about twenty years ago. I did an evaluation of his joints, skin, heart, lungs, and blood and made a pretty easy diagnosis of lupus.

Twenty years later, I have had him maintained with standard lupus therapy. He has never been back to the hospital in twenty years. Frankly, I don't even check his inflammation rates because they don't track with what he's feeling. On random days, they are very high, and on other days they are very low. This is typical proof of what I've been saying this whole time: you never treat blood tests; you only treat patients. Plus, diseases do not read books.

I spend a lot of time undoing the poor care of other doctors, even if it's not something that is in my field. For example, I was treating a patient for something totally unrelated, when I noticed a huge lipoma growth on his back. I asked, "What's the deal with that?" According to the patient, he'd had it for years, and no one would take it out. He had a Medicaid HMO, so no one would see the patient. He'd learned to deal with it. I asked if he wanted me to just take care of it.

He said, "You can do that?"

I said, "I can do whatever is medically necessary," and I grabbed a scalpel.

I had to go into this guy's back up to my elbows to get this thing out. It took about two hundred stitches and staples to close him up. When I was done, I had a twenty-pound lipoma in my hands. When stretched out, it spanned four feet long. (My medical assistant can verify.) He was stunned. He said he felt like he could breathe for the first time in a long time.

It's sad; people will suffer for years because they think that there's no option. Once, for example, I saw a patient who had warts all over his fingertips. The smallest one was the size of a jellybean. These were huge warts that inhibited him from using his hands. On at least five of his fingers, the wart was half an inch long, half an inch wide, and standing up half an inch.

He said he'd had them frozen and burned off for years, but nothing worked, and he'd accepted his plight; this is not the Middle Ages. I told him I could help him. He didn't believe me. I grabbed a scalpel and went to work slicing off all of those warts. After that, I cauterized everything. They never came back, and his life was changed forever, for the better.

Just today, there was another sad, horrible case. I obviously was not rushing and spent two hours with this lady. She was first seen in 2018 at the community hospital to the south of me. She went into the hospital with muscle weakness, and the rheumatologist in that community hospital—along with most others—doesn't do hospital consults. Somehow, this woman ended up being on eighty milligrams of prednisone a day for one year, and they didn't know what was wrong with her. After the year, she hadn't improved at all. Frustrated, she decided to get another opinion, and she went to the University Hospital in Philadelphia. She ended up going there *four* times in search of answers, which is indicative of the lack of good teaching and supervision at one of the nation's most reputable institutions. Each time, she was seen by a different doctor. Each time, she got a different diagnosis. Even after talking with her for two hours, I still haven't figured out what her problem is. I can tell you that I immediately took her off of all of her unnecessary medications. I will not give up until I have figured out what's going on and I've given her relief.

Interestingly enough, a prominent physician at the University of Pennsylvania—due to his insecurities—indicated to me that nobody really knows how to read sacroiliac X-rays. At a conference, I ran into a colleague who is a world-renowned expert in spondyloarthropathy, Dr. Mohammad Azad Khan. I told Dr. Khan that I read my own X-rays, and I find that there's more sacroiliac disease than rheumatoid arthritis. He was elated to hear this and asked if I would announce it in the room because he's been trying to make that point for thirty years. I've concluded that Dr. Khan and I are the only rheumatologists that read sacroiliac films properly. Because I find so many of them, I'm afraid of being audited, so I often order an MRI (fear of audit = waste of money) to confirm my results, and there's been 100 percent accuracy so far.

Some doctors think problems are to be expected with age, and these doctors will appease the patients rather than help them. The whole principle that every problem is related to aging is just not true. You can make a huge difference in someone's life if you take the extra time and effort to find a solution, if you really care. However, most doctors don't.

CHAPTER 4
WHY RHEUMATOLOGY KICKS ASS

In the *Annals of Internal Medicine*, circa 1988, there was an article saying that no one should go into rheumatology, because you can make more money in internal medicine with two years less of training.

Over time and overall, the system fails those of us who require it. American medicine is great for the young and healthy and perhaps a yearly checkup. You leave with a smile. Your family doctor collected your copay, received another payment from your insurance company, and told you that you're healthy. You might even get a lollipop! Unfortunately, there are many people with high blood pressure, diabetes, high cholesterol, and other so-called common problems that require them to go to doctors and have testing on a regular basis.

Although there are specialists who treat high blood pressure, diabetes, and cholesterol, many family doctors do, as well. It has been well established that these conditions—whether genetic or related to lifestyle—have standard protocols for a treatment approach. Generally, most people who suffer from these conditions receive at least the minimum standard of care. If they go to a specialist, they may receive better than that.

However, more and more Americans face health issues that are *not* particularly straightforward, like why did a sixty-five-year-old man develop high blood pressure for the first time in his life yesterday? Why did this woman suddenly lose vision in her right eye? Now, all of a sudden everyone is out of their comfort zone.

This is where a rheumatologist comes in. We are particularly adept at thinking through the more complex and less common diseases that might feature a patient's symptoms. For example, hypertension is a feature of vasculitis. Hypertension is also a feature of scleroderma renal crisis. Most doctors would just treat the symptom of high blood pressure rather than digging deeper to figure out the underlying disease.

I have had so many middle-aged patients come to me who report having had a blood pressure of 240/140 for more than a year. More than once, I've been able to diagnose the underlying issue, stop their six blood pressure medicines, and start the one that will actually solve the problem. All's well that ends well? Not quite. How much blood vessel damage did these people sustain before they came to me? How much higher is their risk of heart attack, stroke, blindness, or kidney failure because of their incorrectly treated blood pressure crisis? Why weren't those patients referred to a rheumatologist within a few weeks or a few months? Why were they always referred to either a cardiologist or maybe a nephrologist? Why did nobody think of sending them to a rheumatologist in the first place? Well, this is a failure of our educational system and/or a lack of attention on the part of the trainees. On the one hand, most doctors prefer to refer to people in their circle of friends. On the other, they don't even know who to refer to. So, let me educate you on what, exactly, a rheumatologist does—and why it could save your life.

It is said that everyone needs a good attorney and a good accountant. I'm here to tell you that they also need a good rheumatologist. If a rheumatologist is used correctly, the rheumatologist could be the most important caregiver in the entire healthcare system. That's because a rheumatologist is 50 percent bone doctor and 50 percent internist extraordinaire. Simply put, I'm an internal medicine doctor who takes care of diseases affecting the whole body, compared to specialists like cardiologists, who focus on the heart, or pulmonologists, who focus on the lungs. I focus on connective tissue; therefore, I focus on everything.

I focus on joints, muscles, cartilage, tendons, enthesis, and nerves. Rheumatic diseases may involve all organs over time, or at one time. All, however, seem to involve joints at some time, thus, they're always rheumatologcal, not orthopedic surgeon. The neck can be involved, which can lead to headaches. The lungs' involvement causes shortness of breath or pleurisy.

Cardiac involvement may be pericarditis, endocarditis, or myocarditis. Other organs have frequent involvement. Constitutional symptoms, such as fatigue, lethargy, weight loss, and fever are signs the patient isn't a prevaricator and has infection, cancer, or rheumatologic illness. Patient history is most important, and family members may help or hinder. A great history will give you the diagnosis. Further, I would say, if you haven't figured it out with the history, the other 10 percent of the time, the physical exam then helps to solidify a diagnosis, which allows for proper laboratory blood tests and X-rays to confirm your diagnosis. Nine times out of ten, the diagnosis is obvious to me just from speaking with the patient.

Simultaneously, I cover the involvements of different diseases that are either attacked by antibodies or that infiltrate the body by substances such as proteins or fats.

Which common diseases are the domain of a rheumatologist? I cover tendinitis (yes, rotator cuff too, so don't see a surgeon, see me), bursitis, enthesopathy, arthritis (and meniscus tears) of a joint. I have expertise with psoriatic arthritis, reactive arthritis (Reiter's syndrome), ankylosing spondylitis, Crohn's disease, polymyalgia rheumatica, giant cell arteritis, rheumatoid arthritis, lupus, Sjogren's, scleroderma, sarcoidosis, inflammatory myopathies or muscle weakness. Joining the hit parade lately are auto-inflammatory conditions and IgG4-RD (related disease). In fact, today I diagnosed aortic involvement in a patient with this disease. With steroid and Rituxan, he should be fine. Vasculitis, which may have protean manifestations in the small, medium, and large vessel, and examples include ANCA vasculitis, PAN, and giant cell arteritis (large vessel).

Sometimes, there are conditions that are much rarer. On two separate occasions, for example, I diagnosed polyarteritis nodosa (medium-vessel vasculitis) in patients walking in the office door. One of the patients subsequently went to a teaching hospital of a prestigious university, only to have the megalomaniac physician at the Ivy League institution refuse to agree with me but agree he couldn't find a better conclusion. (It must suck to be a department chair in the Ivy League and know there is a community doctor who is better at diagnosis and has no students doing his research!) This was the same doctor who disputed my ability to read sacroiliac films. They were motivated to keep that patient at their institution and keep their payments, too.

In the case of the polyarteritis nodosa (PAN), they each went for second opinions because this is such a rare disease, and I encouraged that. However, I cautioned them to remember that a different opinion is not a correct opinion. Even if someone gets eight opinions, the first opinion is frequently the correct one. It's hard for people to accept at times. Sorry, it's a fact.

Unfortunately, in rheumatology, diagnosing does often come down to opinion, in a sense. The diseases that we treat frequently do not have a test to confirm them. Instead, the diagnosis is based on the history, the physical, the clinical presentation, and the exclusion of other conditions. Often, they are based on the utilization and response to treatments, as well. We are constantly weighing a risk/benefit ratio when it comes to deciding on treatment and prescriptions. One of the most challenging aspects of rheumatology is explaining to an intelligent patient that they have a condition but do not fulfill the criteria for that condition. One must understand research criteria are merely there to have a patient enrolled in a research study; however, they are not meant for diagnosis of disease. This is difficult to understand yet exploited by payers and pharmacy benefit managers. They feed off it, so they do not pay for medications unless a patient fulfills criteria that they insist upon—not what is reality. This is one of the reasons people do not always get treated properly. (We all shake our heads when appropriate drugs are denied.)

That's why it's so impressive that I can do what I do. I'm like the Dr. House of rheumatology, minus the pill problem. Honestly, patients often get angry when I diagnose them on the first visit. They're so used to getting the runaround from other milquetoast medical professionals that when they come across someone actually doing their job, something feels off and they think they're getting scammed.

It's even worse if some other doctor has told them "the blood test says" something about their health. Patients think that there's something special about blood tests, that they are truly omnipotent. They are fixated on blood tests. Indeed, blood tests are the reason why many people end up in my office! Somebody unnecessarily orders a blood test that turns out positive for something, and then it needs to be sorted out. Sure, the blood test *might* end up being related to the real problem. Ultimately, however, it's the history that really matters.

If I take a patient's history and I find that there was no reason to order a blood test in the first place (this is what I call pretest probability), I'll tell the patient. In some cases, I can even reassure them that there is nothing wrong, and that they can go off their medication. Sometimes the medication was causing the abnormal blood test in the first place! More often than not, surprisingly, they get angry and even argue with me. We are here to save your life and improve the quality of your life, not to do as you ask, hold your hand, and make you happy at the expense of your health. I have to do what is right by the patients—even if they don't want it.

I'm disturbed to see how often a consultant blindly accepts the conclusions of previous doctors without investigating the data. Doctors should be able to wear many hats, so we can give patients thorough care. We need to analyze our synovial fluids that we obtain, and we should know how to do this better than the pathologist. We should be reading our own X-rays, and we should know better than the radiologist what certain diseases look like and how they are diagnosed by X-ray.

I assure you there is no one alive who can read sacroiliac films better than myself. (Maybe Azad Khan.) First of all, most people don't bother reading them. Second of all, radiologists weren't trained; and third, orthopedic surgeons probably have never even heard of them. I read them for my patients. This is how it works in my office. This is *not* how it works in all offices. I reprimanded an orthopedic spine doctor for removal of inflamed sacroiliac joints, which are easily treated with TNFα inhibitors. This is criminal, in my opinion.

As you can probably guess by now, hospitals are the epicenter of the most twisted treatment that there is, when it comes to these issues. Why? It all comes down to money. Hospitals make a certain amount of money based on how many trainees they have, as well as—obviously—payments for the patients that come through their doors. COVID-19 is a great example: the more of it your hospital sees, the more money you are entitled to. If you show up there with an arthritic flare or a gout flare, they'll treat you. Your wallet and your health will probably be worse off because of it, though.

If people understand that gout is treated by a rheumatologist and should not warrant a hospitalization, this would save them huge amounts of money. I mean *huge*. Your arthritic flares and lupus flares should be managed by a rheumatologist. They should not send you to the emergency room, urgent care, or family physician. If a patient has joint pain—regardless of what they think the cause is—if there was not a trauma severe enough to cause an obvious fracture, thus the lion's share, it is something that should be seen by a rheumatologist. It is truly unbelievable how many patients are treated incorrectly until rheumatology comes along a week later and says, "This is gout. Case closed." Again, huge amounts of money saved.

If patients insist on shelling out for a hospitalization, they're still unlikely to find any real long-term relief. It is almost embarrassing how care is administered at our nation's hospitals. This may be partially due to the fact that patients flock to emergency rooms whenever they have an issue, because they don't know where to go. Patients should understand that going to the emergency room should be reserved for an asthma attack, GI bleeding or pain, trauma, a heart attack, coma, stroke. That does not include joint or bone pain. Orthopedic emergencies include digits that have been accidentally (or maybe not accidentally) amputated, or limbs that have been broken.

All joint pain issues are easily and more correctly treated by a rheumatologist. Even if you have a sprained ankle, the rheumatologist can drain the blood out of the joint to speed the healing process instead of just slapping an Ace bandage on it. (Blood is phlogistic—and needs to be drained out.) We do proper analysis of the joint fluid—known as synovial fluid—to ensure that you don't have a tiny fracture by identifying droplets in the fluid. Proper synovial fluid analysis as reviewed by the rheumatologist can see a fracture before an X-ray is ever done. Neutral lipids can be indicative of pancreatic diseases.

Patients who have chronic pain who fail to see a rheumatologist from the start waste so much money and so many years of their lives. It is mind-blowing to see people with common problems such as rheumatoid arthritis, gout, lupus, scleroderma, Sjogren syndrome, and vascular diseases such as giant cell arteritis be misdiagnosed and in pain for years or even decades.

Yesterday, a doctor called and asked me to see a patient with what he believed to be incorrectly diagnosed shoulder pain. The patient was told by the orthopedic surgeon two months ago that it was a frozen shoulder requiring surgery. So far, he had gone to physical therapy, MRI, three orthopedic visits, and had two injections. When the patient met me, I took a history, and his diagnosis was a diabetic frozen shoulder. The proper injection immediate cured and solved the problem in one second. Hence, that one visit with me would have solved everything. The patient said it was a miracle, and I said it was no miracle all. He just had been treated wrong. The patient was getting worse in physical therapy, which is not uncommon. The physical therapist was following orthopedic directions, but the directions were wrong. I stopped that therapy and stopped his follow-ups. Please realize that I see a jaded population; however, those who just came out of the cast for a broken arm do very well in physical therapy because that would be appropriate use of service.

Why do so many of these shift doctors fail to send their clients to an appropriate specialist—namely, a rheumatologist? In my training, I learned that if I saw a patient who did not respond to the appropriate treatments, the problem was something that should be dealt with by another specialist. (If treatment doesn't go as planned, it's either the wrong diagnosis or wrong treatment,) For some reason, the other doctors do not think of rheumatology as a specialty. As subspecialists, we are probably the least utilized of any specialty.

Generally, hospital-based physicians only think of orthopedics when it comes to joint problems, because they have not been trained adequately—this goes for the referring doctor and the orthopedic surgeon. This could not be a worse decision. They are bone surgeons. I am a bone doctor. A patient shows up to the hospital with a low-grade fever and joint pain, and they are subjected to an unnecessary arthroscopic procedure that will not help the problem. There are *very rare* occasions where these joints are infected, but even in those cases, they can be managed as an outpatient with the joint drained daily and antibiotics administered. (You would prescribe the antibiotics based on what was growing in the fluid, which would best be analyzed by a rheumatologist.)

Instead, I've seen unnecessary amputated digits—fingers and toes—all because of gout attacks that were presumed to be infections. (If someone had used a polarizing microscope to look at the joint fluid, they would be able to identify the gout crystals and prevent the surgery altogether.) I have seen amputations because of diabetic joints that were also thought to be infections. No infection that I have ever seen mimics these rheumatological issues (maybe gout). Moreover, that would be obvious to a rheumatologist as soon as he or she looked through a microscope. (If your rheumatologist does not have a polarizing microscope, you need a different rheumatologist.) In fact, the specimen in the hospital, if not taken by a rheumatologist when sent to pathology, is often in the wrong preservative, which will dissolve the crystals. This is pitiful—like throwing out the specimen! And yes, I have seen that as well! (A dear friend saw his mother die of lung cancer fifteen years ago after three "lost" lung biopsies—her autopsy wasn't. They can't lose an autopsy; that would be as serious as murder in the first.)

How do you know whether to go to an orthopedic surgeon or a rheumatologist? Rheumatologists—who are bone doctors—differ greatly from orthopedic surgeon, who are bone surgeons. Orthopedic surgeons are trained to operate, to see people who are asleep. Considering that 98 percent of injuries do not require surgery, it behooves one to see a rheumatologist first. Rheumatologists who are well trained will be able to find out the cause of your problem, whether it is injury or not. If the rheumatologist—God forbid—finds a bone tumor or a fracture, then on almost all occasions the rheumatologist would refer you to an orthopedic cancer surgeon, like a general contractor referring you to a carpenter.

A less sophisticated rheumatologist I know injected the dreaded Achilles tendon—something that should only be done by the most experienced injector. He caused a rupture, which required major surgery and a year of disability. The point of this story is, only certain people—me being one of them—should be allowed to inject Achilles tendons. If you treat the person properly, and we are not all the same, the outcomes would be better.

I have seen many thousands of patients and seem to have no shortage based on my waiting list. Still, many people don't get it. Let me be clear: if you have shoulder, neck, hand, wrist, elbow, hip, knee, foot, back, ankle, toe, or finger pain, tennis elbow, plantar fasciitis, heel spurs, swelling of the joint, tenderness of a joint, bursitis, tendinitis, or inability to move a joint, you need to start with a rheumatologist.

I'm not trying to say that orthopedics is not important. As a rheumatologist, I do not put casts on broken bones. Nor do I operate and repair tendons; nor do I do joint replacements. These are things that we *do* need the orthopedic surgeons for, and they are important in the treatment of arthritic conditions.

Over the last ten years, the quality of training seems to have diminished. Rheumatology is forgotten because most people are trained so poorly, they don't know what a rheum does; therefore, it all goes to an orthopedic surgeon. An orthopedic surgeon can't do the job correctly. You must hit a bull's-eye 100 percent of the time, and nobody can do that except for me. I have people every day who've been to another rheum or ortho asking me to inject something that was injected two weeks ago because it never worked, and mine works immediately.

Current rheumatology doctors don't have much training in injections, and patients are incorrectly treated and have unnecessary surgery for carpal tunnel, rotator cuff repair, trigger finger release, plantar fascia, and meniscal surgery. I inject it once, and they don't have to have surgery.

For example, a chronically inflamed tendon may rupture. This cannot be fixed without the orthopedic surgeon. However, if this patient had seen me first, the inflammation may not have become chronic or out of control. A bone may die, also known as avascular necrosis, and often must be replaced. A diabetic (Charcot) foot may collapse and need to be fused. These problems all require surgery, which is done by an orthopedic surgeon. However, the initial evaluation for all of these problems *should* be done by a rheumatologist. (If this information comes as a surprise to you, then you need to read this chapter twice.)

What makes me the best at what I do is precision. My injections have saved thousands of people from unnecessary trigger finger, carpal tunnel, rotator cuff, and spine surgeries, and knee replacements. I have done joint injections on people who showed up with Band-Aids on their joints—on the side opposite to where I put the needle. I'd say, "What's that?"

"Oh, well, last week I went to the orthopedic surgeon for the injection," they'd say, "but no more. I'm here to get relief."

"You went to a bone surgeon. Now you want me to fix the problem?"

"Oh, well, my family doctor sent me to the orthopedic doctor," they'd insist. (*You have the right and privilege to tell your doctor to whom you want to be referred, assuming referral is required.*)

I'd reply, "Well, your family doctor doesn't seem to care so much about you. You need to get a family doctor who knows to refer to me first so that you don't have to go get pricked twice and have your insurance double-pay."

"No, I never thought about that!"

Patients don't think about much when it comes to their care; they just do what their doctors tell them. I go ahead and do the shot in the right place with the correct technique. The patients feel much better, they can't believe it. They bring in their friends, their whole family to get treated, and they'll never go anywhere else. I guess the problem is solved.

Sometimes, by the time they see me it's already too late to save them from going under an orthopedic surgeon's knife. I had a patient come in here a week or two ago, and the MRI read, "complete rotator cuff tear." He put it down on the table, and I said, "Hey, let me talk."

He goes, "Look, you know what's wrong."

"No, I don't." I told him. "I haven't talked to you yet."

I talked to him and found that he'd already had rotator cuff surgery, which is almost always unnecessary—unless there was major trauma or a complete full-thickness tear.

He said, "The operation didn't work."

"Well," I said in my smug way, "I think you'll feel a lot better by the time you leave."

He didn't believe it. He said, "I don't know. Those needles hurt."

"You can leave," I told him, "but why'd you come here this morning? To treat it."

I identified that he had inflammation in the tendon of the bicep, which often causes shoulder pain, and I injected him there. I said, "Pull your shirt on."

"No, it's gonna hurt too much."

"Just do it. Does your shoulder feel okay?"

He said, stunned, "It feels completely normal."

The MRI, the red tape, the surgery, none of it was necessary. Nothing worked until I actually talked to the patient to figure out the problem. The patient was cured.

Another patient who came to me went through an even worse travail at the hands of her orthopedic surgeon. This patient told me she had lupus and that she was getting a manicure, and the lady did something to her cuticle and she got an infection. So, she called an orthopedic surgeon, who believed it was an infection, and they cut her open. They thought they saw pus, so they irrigated her arm all the way to the elbow.

The good news is that eventually she made her way to me before they messed her arm up even further. I took a look at the patient, and I said, "You know, I don't know who labeled you with lupus. This looks like a scleroderma case to me." She didn't believe me, but I looked carefully at the lesion and the surgical site. People with limited scleroderma get calcium deposits (hydroxyapatite) under the skin. That's what was in her arm—not pus. There is no treatment for them, and they don't really obstruct a patient's life that much. She didn't need to have her arm sliced open over it. All of the cultures were negative, so everything bad that happened to her was the fruit of a poison tree.

Why are there such problems? It's because we have around 4,000 rheumatologists in the US, and ten times the number of orthopedic surgeons. People wanting to learn rheumatology get limited exposure because of lack of knowledge by their teachers.

This other guy came to me, and he'd been told by an orthopedic surgeon that he needed carpal tunnel surgery. In carpal tunnel surgery, somebody cuts open your hand and removes the transverse ligament that covers the median nerve. What people often don't realize is that carpal tunnel syndrome can have hundreds of different causes. Pregnancy is even one of them! Another common cause is gout, which is one of my favorite conditions to treat. In this case, my investigation revealed that it was caused by hypothyroidism. A normal thyroid function should give someone TSH levels somewhere between 0.5 and 4.5. This man had TSH levels at eighty. He definitely didn't need to get his hand cut open, like his orthopedic surgeon wanted to do. Believe it or not, the surgery was actually done a *second* time in the hopes of getting it right. All that he needed the whole time was treatment for his underactive thyroid. Poor guy had two unnecessary surgeries and has a drain in place that isn't needed. All due to laziness or incompetence.

Yet another horrifying example: lupus patients frequently get fluid around the heart. The treatment for that is steroids, but when they don't call rheumatology, it's a disaster. Instead, they call a cardiothoracic surgeon to cut a pericardial (the lining of the heart) window and let the fluid out. Little do they know, the fluid will probably come back the next day—and the day after that, and the day after that, and so on. Doing that is no different from popping a blister. You didn't fix or heal anything. The way you heal this is with an anti-inflammatory—not cutting a hole in the lining of your heart.

How could those patients have known that a rheumatologist should have been their first call? How can anyone know if their family doctor is making the right choice for them, when no two doctors are equal? Their experience from their training—which you as the patient will never know—guides the decisions that are made. Or, the decisions are made because of doctors simply valuing their friendships, politics, or any number of other reasons that put patient care in last place. When do you need to opt for a rheumatologist?

It all boils down to the fact that everything does end up involving the lining of the joint (synovium). So, I inject joints with what the lay person refers to as cortisone. A simple injection can prevent these unfortunate people from getting unnecessary surgeries, but it's all about the precision, the technique, the experience, and the confidence of the person giving the injection—namely, me. Luckily for my patients, there is no one who can do it better. Not in any field, not in any city, not in any state, or country. People wait in line. I've done hundreds per hour. Both spine and knee. Overall, I've done more than three million injections in my career. How do I even know that? I've bought all the needles from the same distributor. Three million needles, three million injections. Once, I did two knees simultaneously— one needle in each hand. It's very important to note that the injection has to be put in the exactly correct spot, however. I'm not just a beast when it comes to numbers; I'm a sharpshooter.

I am so good at giving injections that I developed tools to make it easier for others. I patented a bent needle called the J Needle to make the whole process more efficient and more comfortable for my patients (Patent #D876619; February 25, 2020). This is just one of the nine national and international patents that I have developed through my company, Jasperate. The company is now for sale, because I want to focus my attention on helping patients.

Jasperate, founded by me, and funded by crowdfunding, is a collection of intellectual property to produce less-expensive needles that are more user-friendly. There is even a kick-ass dialysis needle that will revolutionize dialysis as we know it today. There is a delivery system for medications to be injected in the pleural space. Those companies that produce or manufacture needles need to contact me or my partner, David Weksel, to discuss terms of sale.

In my career, I have been the doctor for my swim team, and I have treated virtually every member of my swim team. I have been the doctor for many other groups and organizations including companies with three hundred to four hundred employees. In my tenure as the occupational physician at a glass company of five hundred employees, there was only one lost-time injury in twelve years due to my diligence. People would pop in for stitches occasionally and simple medical procedures, but nobody had a lost-time injury except for one man who fell through a manhole cover. He actually did require shoulder surgery for his SLAP tear, and he fully recovered due to the work of an amazing orthopedic surgeon.

The San Francisco Giants of the seventies and eighties actually had a team physician who was a rheumatologist, not an orthopedic surgeon. This is a smart trend. Larry Bird's career was ended by psoriatic arthritis, but how long did it take before he was sent to a rheumatologist and treated properly?

Years ago, people were starting to get it, and there was a push for what was called rheumatology primary care. While I don't believe this is necessarily a good thing, I do believe that patients with a rheumatic disease should receive all their care from a rheumatologist, as most of their subsequent health problems relate to their rheumatic disease. Patients should trust the rheumatologist to get to the root of the problem in a way that other doctors can't or won't. For example, many specialists take weekend courses and get a certificate that says that they understand and know how to diagnose and treat osteoporosis. However, in rheumatology, it is part of the basic curriculum. We know this information inside out and backward, and you cannot learn that at a weekend course, or you will simply be the broken clock or the blind squirrel—right twice a day and sometimes stumbling upon a nut.

Most people go to a doctor's office with back pain that will typically go away on its own, so they end up thinking that the doctor was correct in whatever they prescribed. But if something more challenging walks in the door, that's when the men and boys become separated. Asking the right questions is only possible if you understand the natural history of the disease process and how to interrogate like a professional interrogator. In reality, doctors don't need to know what the treatment for anything is, because you can look it up. The most important thing is finding the correct diagnosis, and this is what is lacking. Very few find the correct diagnosis. Very few explain to the patient that in certain instances, finding the definitive diagnosis may take years, or may be impossible.

If you can't diagnose it and you're a great interrogator, it's probably not something in your field. A truly excellent clinician, however, is somebody who can recognize *any* condition, whether they've actually seen it in the past or not.

I have seen very many conditions, including things rare enough to be sent to the NIH (National Institute of Health), where they do genetic mapping to try and determine which rare condition a person has. I believe I can recognize nearly everything within my field and a fair amount in other specialties. (I'm still searching for Gaucher's disease.) Sorry to disappoint, but at the time of this writing, I have just recently done genetic testing and found my first patient with Gaucher's disease. The clue was the deficiency in beta glucosidase, checked because of clinical suspicion. To keep it realistic, I've never seen MAS (macrophage activation syndrome). My best description would be a cytokine storm in lupus or stills. I haven't seen 100 percent of the rheum text, but very close!

Even conditions that are considered rare to any specialist other than rheumatologists show up in my office with some regularity. One example is polymyalgia rheumatica, which is a disease typically of elderly white people. It's similar to rheumatoid arthritis, except it involves large joints and what we refer to as the proximal girdles: shoulder and neck, low back, buttocks, and hips. Most doctors have not even heard of it, but I've diagnosed a case once a week for my entire career.

Even more common than that, though, is rheumatoid arthritis. Two percent of the population or three million people suffer from rheumatoid arthritis, commonly known as RA. Of those, the ratio of women to men is about three to one.

I have been a doctor for many years now, and when I first started in rheumatology, the treatment for rheumatoid arthritis included mostly NSAIDs, oral or injectable gold, Plaquenil, prednisone, sulfasalazine, and penicillamine. These have mostly fallen by the wayside. They were referred to as DMARDs (disease-modifying antirheumatic drugs), which is actually a misnomer, because they don't modify the disease. (Methotrexate is still the #1 drug for RA, and it's a DMARD.)

We are in the era of biologics—large molecules from biologic sources, too large for pills, and destroyed by stomach acid (also known as biologic DMARDs), spearheaded by TNFα inhibitors, interleukin inhibitors, B cell depletion, T cell costimulation. (Although, for interleukin-1 and interleukin-6, interleukin 12/23, interleukin-17a,17f, or B cell depletion, we still use methotrexate and steroids, but less so.) These biologic DMARDs, unlike the previous DMARDs, actually do modify the course of the disease. NSAIDs, gold, and penicillamine are largely obsolete, and thank goodness for that. Much of what I have said for rheumatoid arthritis overlaps with all the spondyloarthropathies by and large.

Drugs in the TNFα category include Remicade (Infliximab) and Enbrel (Etanercept). For interleukin-1, we have Ilaris (Canakinumab) and Anakinra (Kineret). The interleukin-6 drug is Tocilizumab, a.k.a. Actemra. The B cell depletion drug is Rituxan (Rituximab), and it is Orencia (Abatacept) for T cell stimulation.

Much has changed for those suffering. Thirty years ago, the disability rate for rheumatoid arthritis was 35 percent. Now it is minimal if treated early—my estimate is 0.1 percent. If someone comes to me for the first time with twenty-five years of untreated disease, they will not do well. If I'm seeing patients within days, weeks, months, or even a year of their symptoms' onset, however, they do great on the biologic therapy. There are more than six drugs available, when the first three were completely sufficient, in my opinion. I have no idea why the others were developed at all.

There's yet a third class of drugs called small-molecule DMARDs, or JAK-STAT inhibitors. JAK stands for Janus kinase inhibitor. The Janus kinase is a pathway of inflammation. JAK inhibitors already have four different kinds of subgroups that encompass many medications, both on the market and in development. Many delusional researchers and clinicians seem to think that they're the silver bullet we've been waiting for when it comes to rheumatoid arthritis. I completely disagree.

These drugs will not stand the test of time. They do not offer any significant benefit beyond any currently available treatment for rheumatoid arthritis and are loaded with side effects. They are very dangerous and will ultimately kill more people than they save. This is just my speculation, but I believe the writings on the wall. I am not certain why JAK inhibitors are used, and I'm not even certain why they are available. I do think the concept of topical JAK inhibitor is of interest, but so far there has been no novel benefit.

There are now enough drugs to treat rheumatoid arthritis, and spondyloarthropathies. The only way to improve would be to find a more novel approach to the underlying cause so we could produce a medication or gene therapy that would halt and destroy the disease 100 percent. Anything else will be a waste of money on the part of the pharmaceutical industry. Almost all patients can be treated very well with the available medications—provided the insurance companies don't hinder our ability to prescribe them, due to the expense. The cost is really not that shocking when you consider how many people can avoid hospitalizations or unnecessary surgical procedures when their RA is properly controlled. Unfortunately, the insurance companies don't always factor that into their financial equations. We have so many biologics. We need to stop making biologics and focus on developing more treatments for Alzheimer's, brain cancer, etc.

It's become habitual—and more so without the proper training and rheumatology shortage—that all teaching centers will refer their joint problem patients to orthopedics for aspiration, but once the orthopedic drains it, they don't know what to do with it. They're not factoring in the fact that I can do everything better than any orthopedic surgeon when it comes to joints. I'm not just saying it in this book. I'll tell it to their faces, too. I went to an orthopedic meeting and proudly said, "How can all of you make a living operating on joints and think that you can treat joint diseases on a level of quality comparable to that of a rheumatologist? If there were no manpower shortage, orthopedic surgeons might need second jobs." Those people will be working for me some day. I imagine it's possible to make millions of dollars in all specialties, and still make people's lives better. To find out how, read on.

CHAPTER 5
HOW TO BE THE BEST

Choosing a career in medicine opens up many paths. You might be a researcher writing articles and white papers, a politician, or the CEO of a hospital or pharma company. You might be a professor or some kind of academic physician. You may mix clinical practice with academic practice. The list goes on. Truly rising to the top, however, requires that you be self-employed and marry your career. It is the only way to have freedom, liberty, and $$$$$ (not billions). There is no shortcut.

Yet why do some practices thrive, and other practices fail? First of all, these large medical groups and organizations of doctors form out of weakness. Those people aren't strong enough to go out on their own. To have your own practice, you really have to strive for it. With proper training, desire, and a hard work ethic, nothing will be able to stop your bright light from shining, bringing in patients like moths to a flame. You start with a loan from the bank! (I've been told I'm a beacon of shining light in *the sea of darkness that is our healthcare system*.) Nothing can prevent you from doing virtually unlimited work.

To keep patients coming, you must have a strong support network within your office. You must work hard and never look at the clock. You must never say no to a patient, whether they are rich or poor, whether they are kind or rude, whether their insurance is good or bad. (You never know when that nasty uninsured patient may leave happy and send you twenty referrals that have great insurance!)

It costs nothing to smile, be polite, and proudly help people. Exude confidence and people will feel safe in your hands. People love it when I tell them I'm the best—even more so, when I live up to it.

That is a formula that works. Out of enormous masses of patients, our retention rate is higher than ninety-five percent. Thousands of positive reviews exist about me. (My negative reviews include the fact that they didn't like the food that was served in the waiting room.) A large percentage of people thank me for saving their lives. They send me letters saying that I found a cancer that nobody else did, and now they will live. They tell me they would have been crippled with pain without me. Sometimes, someone will post a gushing review on my Facebook page, and I don't even remember treating them! In short, we have made a legendary practice with hard work and skills—skills that only could have been achieved by hands-on training. (Thank you, Bruce Hoffman, and the famous, now-deceased H. Ralph Schumacher Jr.) My practice sees children as well as adults. (Thank you, Don Goldsmith.)

I was lucky enough, years after finishing my own training, to have an old mentor, Dr. Larry Leventhal, experience and evaluate my practice firsthand. Dr. Leventhal had a hand in my training during my years at the Philadelphia VA, and we remained friends in the years after that. After I had been in practice for a few years, I paid him to come down to Vineland and run my practice for a week so I could go on vacation. I don't think he knew what he was getting himself into!

Here's what Dr. Leventhal has to say about what he found when he came to Vineland:

> I was in academics at the time at University of Pennsylvania, and I had four vacation weeks per year. If I didn't use them, I would lose them.
>
> I said, "You know what, Steve? Why don't you go away? I'll use one of my vacation weeks and I'll come down and cover your practice. You'll pay me. I'm not Mother Teresa here. You'll pay me for the work that I do, but I'll cover your practice."
>
> I went down there, and I was amazed by the complexity of patients that he saw and the volume of patients that he saw. I would

come home completely exhausted because he saw so many people. He had to, because it was an underserved area. At the time, I think he was the only rheumatologist in that whole South Jersey area. (Now Soloway = SoJo rheumatology.)

I was beyond impressed with his operation. He had set up a very organized medical facility that had everything in place, and everybody did what they were supposed to do.

I did another week of coverage for him, a year or two later, and then I said, "Steve, I can't do this anymore. It's too exhausting, you know?"

Dr. Leventhal told me that my practice saw more pathology than they see at University of Pennsylvania at any given time and adheres to the same or higher standard of care. Like I said, I learned a lot in training! What was great about that feedback is here's a guy who's kind of like a peer. At that time in my career, even though it was early, most people were thinking everything I was doing was bullshit and financially motivated—that I was just the horror of the system.

Larry comes along, and he's the chairman of medicine and rheumatology at Graduate Hospital in Philadelphia for twenty years. He's a guy who's highly academic and did his rheumatology fellowship at Penn. He was a protégé of famed rheumatologist Ralph Schumacher, and he spent more time with Ralph than I did. (Those of us who were trained by Ralph, we look at ourselves as better than everyone else.)

Larry says, "Steve, every day I saw three people on Cytoxan, how do you manage these people? You're phenomenal. I wouldn't change anything. You're doing everything perfect."

I'm lucky to have known Dr. Leventhal and the rest of my mentors, because you need to have had extensive hands-on training in order to run a successful practice. You cannot do it on book learning alone. Textbooks teach one thing, and then you get out in the world and realize it is not always the same. Of course, textbooks teach the facts of life and the anatomy that exists in 99 percent of human beings. They explain the mechanisms for breathing air in and out, exchanging blood with oxygen, converting food to stool and urine; these things will never change. However, the reality is that diseases do not read textbooks. Textbooks are outdated by the day they are published. If you try to diagnose patients by the book, you'll be making a lot of wrong diagnoses.

Insurance companies must realize for effective medical care, medicine is not a cookbook style, particularly in a highly complex field. It is not possible to operate a practice when, on any given day, you will see any number of diseases, as many as two hundred possibilities or more, that can present to you in two hundred variations or more.

When people come to my office, they often have six things wrong with them, and it is not always easy to connect the dots. Many of them are being treated for some constellation of symptoms that does not have an official name. To treat the patient, though, the insurance company insists on an official name for their issue, even when one does not exist. You must pigeon-hole everyone if you want to be allowed to treat them. How stupid is this? How many people have to be incorrectly treated or diagnosed because the insurance company insists on a name when no name is available? I can tell you for sure that in such a field as rheumatology, this is more common than not. Many people have an enormous number of problems, starting with pain or rash, weakness or inflamed muscles. Complicating things, their blood is normal, even when ordered correctly.

If the blood test is normal, does this mean the patient is lying? Does this mean that they are a drug seeker who should be denied treatment? Of course not. Most patients aren't even looking for pain relief; they are just looking for relief, period. If you can't diagnose them by the book, it doesn't mean that they aren't sick. It means that we as a medical society are not smart enough to test for everything that people can get, so we treat these people symptomatically to ease their suffering even just a little. It's not a long-term cure.

I diagnosed a man with a blood pressure of 240/100 with an anxiety disorder. I stopped six blood pressure medicines and controlled his blood pressure with an anti-anxiety medicine, merely from his history.

I take the time to figure out patients' real problems, even when no one else will. That—combined with my sparkling personality, of course—is what sets me apart in my field and keeps my practice booming. In fact, pretty much the only complaint that I've ever heard from patients is that the wait times are too long. Long waits are inevitable, because I actually spend time talking to patients. (I try to make up for it by ordering gourmet sandwiches and pizza to the waiting room over lunchtime.)

Yet when people remain frustrated with long waits, I simply remind them that they probably have seen ten doctors over ten years to no avail. The four hours they waited for me could have been done ten years ago. Therefore, how long did they really wait: ten years or four hours? As soon as I walked in and solved their particular problem, they quickly realized that every place they went before me either didn't care or didn't know, or both.

Recently, I saw a gentleman who had been to Aruba on a vacation and developed severe diarrhea for forty-eight hours. Upon returning to the US, that bout was followed by severe arthritic symptoms in his large joints. Definitely, both knees were involved. After eliciting a very detailed careful medical history, I realized that I was the third doctor to see him about this issue: he had been to two orthopedic surgeons, and his family physician. In addition, he went on the computer, put in his symptoms, and diagnosed himself with polymyalgia rheumatica. After evaluating him, I diagnosed him with reactive arthritis.

When he came back for his first follow-up visit, he said that he was so happy, the wait time didn't even bother him too much. I replied to him, "You waited an hour for your family physician. You wasted a day for each orthopedic visit. You spent one day in my office for four and a half hours, of which a whole hour was with me. You were not rushed. You were not scurried along. You had a comprehensive history and physical, and I came up with an answer and a treatment plan that day. You admittedly feel much because of it. Tell me, where did you actually waste your time and where did you go wrong in this process?"

He immediately understood that I was referring to the fact that quality means everything; the cream rises to the top. He came to me and waited because my patients do come from all over the country and the world. It's worth the wait.

What happens when you come to visit me, the very best there is? I walk into the room the same way every single time, no matter who's there. I just assume I don't know anybody—or that everybody's an FBI agent or a politician.

Each time, I walk in with my medical assistant, Denise, unless she's on lunch, in which case I walk in with Tina. Denise has been with me for twenty-two years. (My dad had no turnover in his line of work when he was working, either. Maybe it's a family trait. We keep employees, because we treat them well.)

I'll let Denise explain:

My very first impression when I was hired by Dr. Soloway is my impression of him today: he truly cares about his patients, and he wants the best for them. He wants to ensure that they get proper care.

In fact, he's built a reputation for going above and beyond to do that. We'll have patients come in and say, "I was told I need to see you if I'm going to find out what's wrong, that you're the doctor to see." We hear it almost every day, several times a day. There have been tears of joy in the exam rooms, because the patients are always so grateful when someone finally tells them what is wrong and gives them a path forward.

I remember one case, and he probably doesn't even remember this, but a seventeen-year-old girl came in with a lot of joint pain. Her family had taken her to other doctors to no avail, so they brought her to Dr. Soloway. He ran several tests, and the girl ended up having cancer. Everyone else had missed it. She would have died if he hadn't met her.

Because of stories like that, we have a steady stream of patients. The phone is constantly ringing. He always asks if we're going out of business if the phone seems slow to him. It's a very busy practice, and as long as you do your job, you will not have a problem. He leads his staff by example, by being incredibly hard-working, and caring. He'll stay at the office until 10:00 p.m. some nights, but he makes sure that I go home at five. Dr. Soloway really is an exceptional person to work for.

He even took my husband and me to Hawaii. He was going to Hawaii for work, and I was like, "Oh I would like to go, too!" I was kind of joking, of course, but he was like, "Okay!" We spent three days there, and we did everything that we could possibly do. On the first day, he set up for us to do a tour of the Island, and then the next day, he organized a trip for us to Pearl Harbor when he was at a meeting. We did a catamaran ride, walked around Honolulu, and then got ourselves ready to go home.

I've been working by Dr. Soloway's side for a long time, and I'm not going anywhere.

Denise could probably tell you which shirt I'm going to wear on any given day. She probably knows the social security number of fifteen thousand patients. I mean, she doesn't forget anything. She's a human computer. Denise is one of the few people who's smarter than I am by far, and when I tell her that, she doesn't believe me. She is literally my right-hand woman. She is one of the smartest, if not *the smartest*, people I've ever known.

Denise is always by my side, whether the patient is a man or a woman. I just don't go in the rooms alone, even if I've known the person for twenty-five years. Still, I always lead and have my hand out when I walk in to shake hands with the patients. I say, "Hi, I'm Dr. Soloway. It's nice to meet you." That's all, and then I sit down on my stool. They're usually in a chair, and Denise is behind me on a higher stool entering data in the computer as we talk.

I might say, "Let's start off with me taking a look at your paperwork. Maybe I'll get some clues as to what I can help you with." One of the things we have in the chart is a picture of a skeleton, and we have the patients circle the parts that are giving them pain. I get really basic with them to get the bare facts.

I'll say, "All right, so listen. I understand that you have had pain and stiffness for the past six years (or six months or whatever the time is). I need to get a feel for how your day goes, all right? So, stiffness, swelling, do you have one or both of them?"

Let's say you tell me, "Well, mostly it's different, but I wake up with stiffness."

I'll respond, "Is the stiffness five minutes or is the stiffness like more than an hour?"

If you pause or hesitate, I stop. I say, "Listen. You know what? I'm just going to go down a different list of questions. What time do you wake up?"

"Well, my alarm is set for six. I get out of bed at six fifteen."

"Okay. Tell me, what's the first thing you do when you get up?"

"I pee and then brush my teeth."

"Okay. So it takes you five minutes to pee, five minutes to brush your teeth, and then do you shower or do you go to the gym?"

"I go to the gym and I shower at the gym."

"Okay, fine. After you brushed your teeth, that was five minutes. Were you still stiff?"

"Yeah, I was."

"Great. After you pee, that was five minutes. Were you still stiff?"

"Yes, I was."

I got ten minutes covered where I know you're stiff. Then I'll throw in, "When you're standing, do you take anything? Do you take a Tylenol or Motrin, you know?"

"No, probably not."

"Okay. So, you wake up at six o'clock, and you start your exercise routine at seven, and how far do you live from the gym?"

"Twenty minutes."

"Okay, based on that, you have to leave your house at six forty. Are you stiff when you get in the car?"

"Ah, yes I am."

"Okay, now we've proven you're stiff for forty minutes in the morning, which you probably couldn't have told me if I asked you flat out." We can end that conversation, because I know what I needed to get from you.

On the flip side, you have the people who have another set of conditions. They tell me they get up in the morning, and the first three steps, they limp. By the time they pee and get back to whatever they're doing, though, they forget about the stiffness and they're better. I already know what is going on. I can take a halfway intelligent person and force them to give me the answers I need by asking the right questions. It's like if you want to know if somebody's an alcoholic. You don't ask them, "So, are you an alcoholic?" You want to ask them how much they drink. You might even want to double it.

Once a patient loves me, they'll tell me *anything*—and not just about their medical issues. One guy let it slip that he had seventy kids. (I swear, Denise can confirm this!) He had twins when he was thirteen, and they got married for the first time before he ever got married himself. That wasn't the end of his story, though. He said he'd killed two people, fled to St. Louis, and then finally had come back after he killed somebody in St. Louis. With seventy kids, supposedly he had several hundred grandchildren. I think he had seven or nine wives. He couldn't have made this stuff up if he were on LSD. That one dropped off the face of the Earth, though. I think he's probably in prison.

Then again, there was another guy who had "FUCK YOU" tattooed inside his lower lip, upside down and inside out, like an ambulance. (Not only did he have it tattooed; but rather, he tattooed it in prison himself.) When he pulls down his lower lip, he can say it without saying it: FUCK

YOU. He's currently a "lost to follow-up," as we call patients who don't show up for care. That means he's probably locked up, too.

The prison system is the second-highest payer. You know, if I bill the prison a million dollars for a cupcake, they'll pay two million. That's just how it goes. They're defrauding the government. Yes, I do treat prisoners.

One day we had this guy in an orange jumpsuit, and he was shackled at his hands and feet, everything connected with chains. Plus, there were two guys in the room with guns. Wow. I took a look at the guy, I glanced at the armed correction officers, and I asked the prisoner, "So, what did you do? Did you kill any doctors or anything? Do I need to worry about you?"

This guy, he says no, that he's not violent at all. Looking at his paperwork, I tell him, "It says here you got a thirty-five-year sentence. What do you mean you're not violent? You must be nuts!"

He says to me, like a kid from Brooklyn, "Nah. You know, I'm a good guy. I just sell drugs."

I'm like, "How many fucking drugs do you need to sell to get thirty-five years in prison?!"

He said, "Well, I sold a barge."

A barge. Again, Denise can confirm all of this.

My most daunting patient interaction, though, was not with one of the prisoners. It was just a normal day with a normal patient when I walked into the room, looked at the guy, and told him straight off the bat, "You know, are you aware that you have psoriatic arthritis?"

He flipped out. "Are you a fucking quack?! You didn't even touch me yet."

I said, "I have two eyes. . . . You've got blue jeans on, too. I didn't have to touch you to know you've got blue jeans on."

This guy lost it. He goes, "You're a quack!" and starts swinging punches.

I'm sitting across the room on the stool, and my guardian angel Denise is trying to keep him away from me, knowing that as a physician, I prefer not to hit someone, even in defense.

I told him, "You need to get the fuck out."

Denise put her finger on his nose and said, "You heard what Dr. Soloway said. Get out."

The guy's girlfriend was with him, and she said, "Honey, we've got to go."

There was so much commotion, patients from every room were wondering what was going on as I yelled down the hall, "I'm going to call every rheumatologist in the United States, so that nobody will ever let you in their office. Nobody will see you. Nobody. Nobody will ever treat your psoriatic arthritis, you sorry ass." Never saw that guy again, but it was all so unnecessary. We have about five hundred people with psoriatic arthritis and 100 percent of them are in remission. He lost his chance at relief because of a bad attitude.

By far, that wasn't the only time we had a massive tumult in our office. Sometimes, it can feel like a three-ring circus! Once, there was a woman sitting in a chair in an exam room, under a small nine-inch TV that was strapped on a small metal shelf near the ceiling. The woman somehow noticed that the TV was moving if the door opened or closed. I don't know what possessed her, but she got up and slammed the door—on purpose—so hard that the TV fell off the thing and hit her friend in the leg. She did it but then had the gall to say she was going to sue me.

Another woman fell purely by accident in the hallway, and the first thing she said was, "I'm gonna sue you because your floors are uneven."

I told her, "Thousands of people have walked these floors, and you're the only one who's ever fallen." She never sued.

Overall, my interactions with patients are much more positive. Many of them even end up becoming my close friends. For example, there was a very intimidating motorcycle club member named "Road" who befriended me and took my infant children for a ride on his purple Harley. He was the most venerable member of this old motorcycle club, Wheels of Soul. All these guys have street names; for instance, Gunny. I met him at the gym, and he was one of the nicest people I ever met. People asked me why I talked to him. Why not? He's always nice to me. I mentioned him to Denise, and she said he was the local stickup boy when he was twelve. Next time I saw him, I said, "What's up with your body?" and he said he had been shot four or five times.

Gunny comes to my office when he's not in prison. If he ever has medical problems, I take care of him for free because I like him. He's a nice person.

I love meeting new people and diagnosing them. In fact, about seven years ago I said, "You know, I'm not going to see follow-ups anymore. I'm only going to see new people."

My CEO, Debra Richards, says to me, "OK, so in three weeks when you're out of new people, then what?"

Well, in those three weeks, Debra made a boo-boo. We have a waiting list of hundreds, and we have six thousand follow-ups in the book. Oh my God, it's insane. It's spread out for months. Unless you know someone who knows me personally, or it's an urgent situation, it could take a few months to get an appointment.

Still, seven years later, on Fridays I only see new people no matter what. Even if I have to stay there twelve hours and see twenty people. My favorite part of medicine is lessening the burden of people who are chronically ill. That's why I do what I do.

"Dr. Soloway truly is one of the hardest-working people that I know," Debra says today. "I've worked with him for two decades, and he wouldn't have been able to build the practice that he did from the ground up if he weren't so dedicated. He has put so much into this practice."

Patient flow is stimulating the brain; however, creating convenience with great tenants that become part of your patient care network makes a nice seamless flow. In fact, there's an imaging center, a phlebotomy lab, and administering of IV medications (infusion center) on the premises, which helps me create more community jobs at the same time. We've done this so much, I've lost count.

Doing well was not by accident. A friend at the gym once said to me, "Hey Steve, is it true all doctors make the same amount of money?"

I shot this man a look and said, "Yes, in Medicare for All or in socialized medicine. . . . Of course not. No doctors make the same amount of money.

Nobody's equal." Five different doctors could see the same patient for the same type of visit, and all five doctors would get different amounts of money for it, pending the insurance company and the contract. Insurance companies on the whole are friendly to deal with and congenial with physicians. With them, it's a mutually beneficial relationship, while Medicare offers the unique concept of unilateral loyalty. They offer discounts and specials if you work in an underserved area, but it is on their terms only, not yours.

It reminds me of that old saying from Soviet Russia. In the US, it used to be a day's work for a day's pay. In Soviet Russia, they said, "You pretend to work, and we pretend to pay." With Medicare, it's "You work, and we make it a nightmare." They also are the worst with audits, but we'll get to that later.

When I started in practice, the old timers told me, "HMOs are no good. We used to get paid in cash!" Well, within a short time I was able to adapt to the system. This is where my negotiating skills came in very handy. I was able to negotiate contracts better than anyone else. (This was not by accident. I was able to show the insurance companies how much I could save them by providing good care.)

Commercial insurers were happy that I was saving them money by doing high-volume quality work, in contradistinction to the government model. As more of Medicare's people came, more of their auditors came. It didn't mean I was doing anything wrong; it just meant I negotiated better contracts. All companies negotiate; even the federal government will negotiate on the rarest of occasions. With everyone else, there is a dialogue. There is no dialogue when it comes to the federal government.

When I first moved to Southern Jersey, everybody who participated with Medicare received a 5-to-10 percent bonus because it was considered an underserved area. Well, once the area suddenly became *not* underserved anymore, they made all specialties exempt. I have no idea which metric they actually used. From looking around here, nothing's changed. What's changed is probably that they just don't want to keep paying us money.

The bonus disappeared. Many doctors were furious about this, but at least the government had no problems paying the bills. Since that time, though, the rates to physicians have been cut each year.

Now there is a new hot topic called "surprise medical billing." The government in its infinite wisdom would like to have price fixing across all private insurance companies, which would essentially take away all negotiating abilities between doctors and insurance companies. This would be totally insane. I thought we were a free market society, no? I didn't realize that we are now living in a shadow society of hidden socialism that already exists. (Kudos to President Donald Trump for opposing this!)

If you don't already know, this is just one example of the fact that we do live in a socialist country. We do not have freedom of speech. We do not have freedom of our liberties. People are not created equal; if they are *created* equal, they certainly don't live equal lives. It is very sad that there is such inequality, but there will always be inequality, despite whatever you write on a piece of paper. This is human nature. Some of us are just better than others, and we didn't get that way by scamming or anything like that.

Most doctors are fair, honest, and hard-working. Most old-school doctors didn't have to worry about money, because with hard work they always made good money. Today's doctors seem to expect a big paycheck as soon as school is over and don't realize how much hard work is necessary to get yourself into a position to be constantly busy and sought after.

In a free market society, we would be able to set our own pricing to reflect that. Most doctors are not looking to price gouge. Doctors are not planning to become billionaires. Doctors are merely looking to be treated fairly and be remunerated for the work that they do. They don't appreciate that in contradistinction to the private sector, Medicare is the only system that lowers your salary every year, no matter what you do. To Medicare, success is suspicious. That should tell you something about how the system works. Efficiency and optimal care are so far out of the norm, they raise red flags.

Ten years ago, under the Obama administration, Medicare found a new way to take advantage of doctors. They announced the Recovery Audit Commission, or RAC. Supposedly, they were intended to identify and recover Medicare overpayments. (Overpayment is code for: You didn't put the right words in the chart, therefore, the patient visit didn't occur.)

They hired a third-party contractor to take back my money until they could prove that I actually did the work. However, these losers that couldn't get a job doing something else were looking for basic keywords, and if the keywords were missing, they made the assumption that I never did the work. That was the case even if the patient and the doctor and the medical assistant all acknowledged that a visit took place. They didn't allow for any wider logic. They would take back your money for something as small as a flu shot if they could not understand why the patient was there to begin with. They extrapolated this over years and tried to destroy practices to the tune of millions of dollars. (Not to mention, these contractors got a 20 percent cut of whatever they pulled back, which certainly influenced their decisions.)

The whole thing was a debacle that just ended up punishing good doctors who were managing to make money under Medicare. It was a sneak attack. They would borrow one or two charts, extrapolate the data, and come back and say, "You owe me ten million dollars."

Audits are a perfect way to keep people honest, but the audits should be *fair* across the board. The reality, though, is that people are audited solely based on billing. For people who complain that doctors make too much money, don't worry! The government takes back your money if you're in the top 10 percent of billers. It is simple: the government fears successful entrepreneurs; if you work too much, here comes the government! The auditors do not know how to figure out what they should be looking for, and it's a total waste of time, yet higher-billing docs can be criminalized.

I know this firsthand. It happened to me in the late 2000s, when they came in and told me that Medicare had supposedly overpaid me to the tune of $2.3 million. It was one of the first RAC audits in the United States. After

I spent several hundred thousand dollars in legal fees and appeared in the third district court (the third of five possible levels of appeal), the judge overruled their decision, and I did receive my money back. I spent most of it on the extra staff, accounting firms, coding firms, auditing companies, and other professionals that I needed to go through the audit.

The damage was done. With the economic downturn, the timing couldn't have been worse, and it hurt me very badly.

It was rough, but it wasn't the end of it. Medicare came back six years later for a totally different reason. This time, they said that my notes were too cookie-cutter, and that it was not proper. (How ironic that during one of my audits, the patients were contacted directly by letter, and the letters were all exactly the same.)

It was just a classic example of the stupidity of government bureaucracy. What was I supposed to do? If someone comes to McDonald's for a hamburger, there is really only one way to order and serve a Big Mac. There is pretty much only one way to describe a knee injection. I placed the needle. I injected the medication. The patient went home. It's not that complicated.

When the government comes calling, though, you don't have much recourse. All you can do is go along with it, because you are the one with your license at stake. Without a license, you cannot be self-employed, an employee, or anything. They have endless time and resources to mess with you.

Of course, the big daddy of government stupidity is the IRS. Somehow, when I flew around the country in private jets to treat my celebrity population, the IRS limited me to $4,000.00 per flight and audited back the rest of the money above that. I had never realized that the type of plane I flew was the business of the government. (Not to mention, I gave the IRS photos of me with all of my celebrity clients.)

Frankly, they should be pleased with rather than afraid of me, as a self-employed physician who has thirty full-time employees. Everyone should love me. But instead, the IRS decided to penalize me, solely because they can. They came up with an arbitrary number I should have been operating at, knowing full well that there was complete justification for me to fly private: I needed to serve my patients on the road and return to the practice as quickly as possible to serve the patients there.

Governmental overreach is gravely affecting the private sector. Many physicians now work for hospitals instead of going into private practice. They have broken down in the face of red tape. They sell their practice to a hospital, so the hospital administration can fight the insurance companies tooth and nail and probably win most of the time. Indeed, they can afford it, because the government pays them off. The government would rather audit ten thousand hospitals than a million family doctors. Meanwhile, the doctors' offices close down, the hospitals grow, and so do the problems of the average American patient.

CHAPTER 6
MEDICARE FOR ALL, PATIENT CARE FOR NONE

You'd better believe that's not all I have to say about Medicare—and worse, this idea of Medicare for All. Medicare for All would be a complete disaster. Medicare for some *is* a complete disaster now. It's often said that if a woman is really beautiful, you can overlook that her personality may not always be friendly. If a woman is really nice, you can overlook that she may not necessarily be aesthetically to your liking. Medicare is mean *and* ugly.

Having a Medicare for All system would lead to the end of medicine in our country as we know it. All doctors would be on shift work, and there would be no motivation to work more than your required fifteen minutes per patient. Doctors would be getting up and leaving the room after fifteen minutes, saying, "Sorry, you have to make another fifteen-minute appointment for another time." (By the way, this is already happening with telemedicine.) Americans would be fleeing to Canada, Australia, and European countries for the best care those countries offer—which is still a close second to what we can offer in the United States.

Despite the timeliness of the debate, this issue goes all the way back to the era of Woodrow Wilson (the founder of the New Idea) and Franklin Delano Roosevelt (originator of the New Deal). LBJ sealed the deal with Medicare and Medicaid.

Many capitalists like to slam FDR as the catalyst that started social welfare programs in the United States. To me, however, he was well-intentioned. He just did not imagine how large the government would get, and how corrupt it would become. First, people just don't understand the difference between social *programs* and social*ism*. Second, we vastly overestimated the work ethic of the American people when these programs were conceptualized.

President Truman first called for the establishment of a national healthcare fund in 1945, as World War II was coming to an end. The World War II generation happened to be the greatest generation of all time. The draft took all walks of life, and everybody had one thing in common: they were proud to be an American, and proud to be Made in America. People were so proud to do something as inconsequential as putting on a hubcap. You know, they couldn't have been happier! They were proud of their country, and proud to support it. Therefore, they deserved to have the government's support. It was two-way loyalty. Now, not only have we created a lazy socialist society by giving out free stuff, but we've created career politicians. People despise the country—unless you're a millionaire—and it's not entirely their fault.

Over time, people became greedy. Jobs and production were outsourced. Companies were operating in a manner that was legalized slavery. As much as I am a capitalist, I smelled this coming in the seventies and eighties when all the jobs started going to China and Mexico. I thought, "Well, all these people here are losing their jobs, so they're going to be unemployed." At the same time, LBJ finalized Medicaid and Medicare, creating more opportunities for complacency and laziness.

While many people took advantage of the system, it still wasn't enough to help people who really needed it. If you're a guy living in Detroit who worked hard for twenty years and then got fired, you're not old enough to collect. You can't get a pension. The company's out of business, and when you're sixty-seven, they give you eight hundred bucks a month or a week or whatever it is. It's enough to live in a shed, maybe behind the garage, which might have partially running water and a toilet that doesn't work. It's very sad stuff. Just because some guy who had ten million needed twelve million, he farmed out all his jobs, and he sold out the people of the United States.

As much as there were people—like our friend in Detroit—who needed help, over time all the losers jumped on the bandwagon and took advantage of the system. So now, it's a free-for-all. These people are always looking for handouts, you know? Trump did something really smart. If you want to get Medicaid, you need to do *something*. You need to work a little bit. Lick envelopes or something. That was brilliant, because it makes people accountable to a degree. Trump doesn't give anything away for free. He's all about "Do something to earn something." That's one step toward fixing this broken system.

Most politicians besides Trump are has-been attorneys who want to ride the gravy train for perks, pensions, and insider trading. (That's why you can enter the White House poor but leave with forty acres in Hawaii!) Every few years, they come up with some harebrained idea to drive people to socialism. This is despite the fact that they know very well that unless the universal basic income were ten million dollars per year, socialism would never work in a country as well-off as the United States.

The latest of these losers railing against the system is Alexandra Ocasio-Cortez—the Aggressive Outcast. She says that we clearly have a problem with healthcare in this country because we have forty million people who are uninsured. First of all, there are about three hundred million people who *are* insured. Why are we once again pandering to the pitiful? If something works for 90 percent of the people and fails 10 percent of the people, why are we going to break up the 90 percent that works to assist the 10 percent of people that it fails?

Medicare for All *would* provide access for everyone, but that's not necessarily something that we should want. First of all, access to care is *not* the same thing as access to quality care. In fact, they're very often opposites. Second, not everyone in our country *should* have access to healthcare! I take offense to the idea that the health treatment of illegal aliens should be paid for with taxpayer money, for example. Why anybody might think they should be able to go to the doctor for free without putting in the work makes no sense to me. The guy at the diner doesn't feed you for free, so why should doctors treat you for free?

When it comes to those actually putting in the work to run our healthcare system—the doctors—they are the ones who are already being hurt by the Medicare mess. If we were to institute Medicare for All, more doctors would quit or retire early.

No doctor is happy with Medicare, because Medicare has reduced physician reimbursement for each of the last twenty years. Medicine is the only job in a free market society where you continually work more and make less. It audits the most and causes more overhead expenses. It was taboo to discuss the finances of medicine in the seventies and eighties, but now we understand the economics of medicine, and doctors shape their careers now with more avarice than even before. That's why the standards are getting lower. No one wants to be a doctor if you have to get a second job to get by.

In the old days, it was assumed all doctors made a lot of money. In the new days, people only choose to go into fields where they think they can make a lot of money—and that doesn't include fields that service Medicare. More and more, it will become impossible for anybody to make any money except for self-employed Beverly Hills and Manhattan plastic surgeons. That's because the wealthy will always have money. The middle class will always have to eat. The poor will always have cigarettes, and so they'll always need medical care. This is the sad truth of the bitter cycle. I'd like to see Bernie Sanders on Medicare and find out he has to pay up front and get reimbursed and be hassled like the average normal crowd.

Here is how a doctor gets paid for a typical Medicare patient. If you go to Manhattan or another affluent city, you're going to have a really hard time finding someone who will accept Medicare assignments. Some doctors will see you, but you have to pay the bill yourself. It's called cash pay. Then, you submit the bill to Medicare to get reimbursed. For example, somebody with my skill set would charge anywhere from five hundred to twelve hundred dollars for a new consult in Manhattan. So, the patient pays five hundred or twelve hundred dollars out of pocket. When they submit the bill to Medicare with a receipt, they'll get back one hundred and fifty dollars from Medicare, and the doctor will get five hundred to twelve hundred bucks from the patient. Everybody in Manhattan is either rich enough to pay for the visit and then get reimbursed a third of what they paid, or they simply don't seek proper healthcare.

Well, I don't live in Manhattan. I live in Vineland, New Jersey, and things are less expensive here. My fee for a new consult is four hundred dollars for a cash-paying patient. When I take someone with government insurance, though, I probably get a hundred and fifty bucks. That's less than half of what I can get with cash pay. You can see why most doctors are phasing Medicare out, and they don't want it. When I say that Medicare for All means care for nobody, I mean it.

Even for those who are willing to deal with the lower payment rates, Medicare is such a hassle. In addition to all of the red tape, audits, and government harassment, the newest trick the government has introduced is requiring preauthorization for anything that costs more than a dollar.

Here's how that works—or, how it doesn't. If a patient comes to my office and they want their knees injected, the first time they come is fine. If that patient wants additional treatment, however, such as viscosupplementation—Rooster Comb shots, as they are commonly known—the patient must go to physical therapy first. It's ridiculous. You take a patient with knee pain who needs help, and you make him pay twenty-five or fifty dollars copay per visit for twelve visits at physical therapy (under Medicare Advantage). That costs up to six hundred dollars. Then, if the physical therapy doesn't work (99 percent of patients swear it makes them worse—just how much did the PT lobby pay the feds to get this joke of a deal?), only then can they come to my office and pay more copays just to get the injection that they wanted in the first place.

It's a total rigamarole, and the patients won't stand for it. They're frustrated, instead of going through the whole drama, they'll just go straight to pain management and get Percocet. It's cheaper, faster, and easier. Obviously, it's much worse for them in the long run.

This is reflected in the numbers at my practice: I used to do fifty people, one hundred joints in a week. It wouldn't take long, and everybody was 100 percent better. Now, if I do one a week, it's a lot. People call up and they say, "Hey, the doctor gave me those back shots like three years ago. I need them again."

My staff has to tell them, "You can't just come in for the shots anymore. You have to make an appointment. First, you'll have to be seen. Then, you'll probably need your MRI updated. You need to go to physical therapy. We have to try a trigger point injection. Basically, you're looking at two to three visits, plus physical therapy and all the copays that go with that."

You can see why such a patient would think getting a prescription for oxycodone or something like that would be easier. They take the easy way out and end up just taking pain pills forever.

When we do manage to eke out a living, Medicare is so shocked, they launch the audits. Someone says, "How can you possibly do such high volume?" (See words of Dr. Leventhal.) Hello: it's because I'm working so hard. I'm sorry, but there's a guy working at Goldman Sachs getting eight hundred thousand dollars a year, with a bonus of twenty-five million. Why shouldn't I push to see as many patients as I can? They make me feel almost criminalized for working hard.

To the auditors, the highly prolific nature of my practice—which is due to my fine skills and high efficiency—is impossible to understand. One time, I actually had a Medicaid investigator come out with a badge. He said, "I want to see where you give the infusions. He looked at the room and he left. I said, "Sir, what were you here for?"

He goes, "A fraud audit."

I said, "Well, what's the audit about?"

He says, "Well, I had to check that you actually are giving the drug. Sometimes we send money to a mailbox for reimbursements and there's no practice there at all."

Bureaucrats are good at auditing, but they can't understand a day in the life of a doctor like me. Ultimately, though, they don't care to understand. It's all about money and them trying to take back what they pay out.

What they don't realize is that the doctor is not the problem in the system. There is money wasted everywhere, and the doctor is getting the least of it. Meanwhile, hospitals and urgent care centers get paid exorbitant amounts of money by creating unnecessary bills and cutting corners. For them, making money comes above patient care. I have seen hospitals switch from using a heparin flush to a saline flush—even though the heparin can prevent blood clots in the patient. That is so wrong, but there's nothing I can do about it.

For most other doctors, it's not worth it. More and more, they're turning fifty and retiring so they can escape all of the red tape, auditing, and harassment. This is going to create the greatest shortage of doctors in the history of our country if this continues.

It will be a total disaster, and who will replace them? I'm sorry, but there is no nurse practitioner (NP) capable of filling the shoes of a subspecialist. (I trained a nurse practitioner better than most rheumatologists practicing today.) How can even the best physician extender—an NP or physician's assistant—know as much as a subspecialist who did five years of residency? Nurse practitioners don't do residency, so where can they fill in that gap of first-hand knowledge? How is it even fair for them to see the complicated cases when they have so much less education than a doctor?

A good nurse practitioner could be a triage nurse, but not more than that. I personally have trained dozens of nurses in my specialty, and after an hour working with me, they all realize one thing: how little they know. That's not meant to be an insult. They readily admit how poor their training was. They don't learn anything useful until they get to a place that actually serves ill people, instead of the system.

Could socialism be the answer? We're heading that way, if we're not there already. Socialism and communism take root when the lowest guy on the totem pole cannot feed his family, and the system collapses. Those in power change the language, change the communications, keep the rank and file stupid, make sure everyone gets a piece of bread, and the people who are running the party are running away with your money.

If you're Joe Blow living in a society like that—say, Saudi Arabia or China or Russia—you're dirt poor. You're garbage. You're nothing. You have nothing.

You eat crumbs. Meanwhile, the oligarchs sell oil. The oil brings in three or four trillion dollars. Somehow, the way their tax system works, they're left with 99 percent of the money. They share that with their friends and family, and the other billion or so people are fighting over a donkey in a burning pile of garbage. That's okay for the oligarchs, because when the poor die, they get replaced. I mean, in China if you're not needed, you may just disappear.

As you can see, socialism is a great system as long as you are a socialist leader. I imagine communism is a wonderful thing, too, if your name is Vladimir Putin. The same goes for the Saudi oligarchs. Still, it's a disaster for the normal people who live within it.

As a real-life example, I want to share the story of one of my friends who lives in England. This woman has had severe swelling in both arms and legs for three months. She went to the hospital and was told that it wasn't a feature of coronavirus, so she needed to go home and call her general practitioner. Her GP is closed because of the coronavirus, so she has to find out through the National Health Service who is taking his place. Turns out, there is only one doctor taking his place, and he only takes phone calls at certain times. This guy tells her he will call in a one-week prescription for water pills for her swollen legs. He will not evaluate her because he does not have to. She cannot go to the hospital because they will not take her. She needs a full evaluation of the deeper problem, not just treatment for her symptoms. That's just one example of why socialized medicine is lousy. Medicare for All is socialized medicine and is also total crap.

Assuming we *don't* want to go down that road, what should we do?

What about going back to focusing on HMOs? Roughly thirty years ago, everyone was complaining about HMOs, because HMOs required patients to get referrals from their gatekeeper-type doctor. It was an adjustment, but everyone adopted and adapted well to that system. Frankly, that system worked quite well and always has.

Barring that, Medicare and Medicaid, the VA, and Tricare (military) should be lumped together as one, and the VA health system as we know it should be closed permanently.

There are one hundred million people who are costing the government ten thousand per year per person for healthcare. Those people are mostly elderly (Medicare-age). Then, there's two hundred billion dollars assigned to twenty million people for the VA. However, only thirteen million veterans are actually using it (free prescription, eyeglasses, hearing aids). Lumping them together would allow you to save seventy million dollars, which would allow you to add thirteen million people to my NEW Medicare, without spending any money. Overall, that would lower the number of uninsured to twenty-seven million.

Second, they need to stop the rate cuts. That's not where money's being lost or wasted. It's being lost and wasted by people double-dipping. You shouldn't be on Medicare if you already have VA insurance, and vice versa. You shouldn't be using Medicare if you already have private health insurance, too. I mean, when I turn sixty-five or sixty-seven, I'm assuming I'll still be working. My primary health insurance is going to be the Blue Cross that I buy now, but the government is going to force me to take Medicare, too. I don't even have the option to not have it! In that sense, we already are living through Medicare for All.

People don't realize that we *are* living in socialism. It's just not as extreme here yet. The only people exempted from that system are the richest: people who have enough money for extremely expensive insurance plans, or those who can afford to pay cash for everything. Honestly, more and more people are doing just that.

The Democrats issued in this new era of socialism lite ten years ago, when they decided that we needed to expand healthcare and involve the government. Prices started to rise. Insurance companies started to deny all testing. Testing could not be done at all if it was expensive.

In fact, I once was on the phone speaking with an agent from Blue Cross on behalf of a patient. I was arguing that an MRI was needed for a particular situation, but it kept getting denied. When I asked what to tell the patient, the rep said they should get better, more expensive insurance, and then they could allow the test. Well, I felt uncomfortable telling the patient this. I went back to the patient and simply stated that the company would not budge and that hopefully we could write an appeal.

In various cases like this, patients become frustrated and they give up. They skip follow-up appointments, they don't take care of themselves, and then they wind up getting admitted to the hospital. In the end, the bills are much larger. The system has become penny-wise and dollar-stupid.

That's the sad reality of every system we have ever tried in our country. The greed of one half of the country and the laziness of the other leaves us with a system that costs too much for everyone.

In sum, issuing universal healthcare to American citizens would be like issuing driver's licenses. Nearly everybody can get one, but that doesn't mean everyone can afford everything else that it takes to drive. (Now they're even giving them to illegal aliens!) Those who can afford it will always take a limo or a private jet. Everyone might get healthcare, but some of us are getting the McDonald's version, and some are getting the Michelin-starred restaurant in Dubai. I know which one I want.

CHAPTER 7
THE VA IS FUBAR

I don't get why there is so much commotion about veterans and their healthcare, or why we still have a Veteran's Healthcare Administration at all. Sadly, it is a huge example of government waste.

In fact, President Trump once said, "for every regulation made we need to get rid of two other regulations." Well, since he created the Space Force, I think we should have to get rid of another major defense program, and that would be Veterans Affairs.

I spent one year in the Philadelphia VA in the late 1980s. To call the place a joke would be a compliment. The first thing I noticed walking in the door was President Reagan's portrait. Next to President Reagan's portrait was a big sign that read, "Your personal phone calls cost this institution $139 million dollars a year."

Fraud, waste, and abuse were rampant within the VA, starting with the phone call issue. People would press nine to get an outside line, and there were no restrictions beyond that whatsoever. Everyone from personnel to patients and even doctors were calling overseas for hours at a time, calling nine-hundred numbers for hours at a time, running up tremendous bills. The VA was smart enough to catch that, and bothered enough to make a sign about it, but they weren't smart enough to block nine-hundred numbers and overseas calls to begin with. It was like money flowing out on the phone wires every day.

Drugs were rampant, too. If you wanted to buy drugs like cocaine, you could go to the VA, where they knocked out the drop ceiling at night and traded money for drugs.

The people who worked there were government employees and couldn't be fired, so they didn't really care what went on. None of it was frowned upon—even if it hurt the patient. Patients went to the PX to steal merchandise and sell to staffers or students or anyone! Anyone who knew the lunch cashier got free food. If it wasn't nailed down, it went to the first undocumented shopper.

Luckily for me, I didn't have to depend on the VA staff for training and expanding my medical knowledge. My mentor at the time was an incredible professional, Dr. Larry Leventhal of UPenn. Our time together was invaluable. I'll let him describe it:

> When I was an attending physician at the University of Pennsylvania, one of the institutions that we covered was the Philadelphia Veterans Administration Hospital, and Dr. Soloway was rotating there when I met him.
>
> The VA had students from UPenn as well as the Medial College of Pennsylvania. Steve always loves when I say that he was much more into it than his Ivy League counterpart. No matter what work needed to be done, he was always there to do it. He would do *her* work if she didn't want to do it.
>
> He always asked a lot of questions and always wanted me to teach him how to do a procedure. He was hungry for knowledge, and as a teacher, you love having students who love to learn and are passionate in that way.
>
> We used to have this little plastic carousel where the consults would be held. There was a compartment for him and a compartment for the other fellow. Steve would do his, but the other fellow would never pick up hers. Steve said, "Well, she's not doing hers. Can I do them?"
>
> I said, "Yeah, just get them done."
>
> He would do both his *and* her consults, because he wanted to get exposed to as many patients as possible and to learn as many procedures as possible. That's the kind of student he was.
>
> The fact that he had gone to a Caribbean medical school didn't make a difference. If anything, I think he used that as a chip on his

shoulder to prove that he was as good as or better than everybody else. He was fueled by that desire.

Another of his mentors, Dr. Bruce Hoffman, and myself always appreciated that willingness to go above and beyond. We would always tell him that you can't go overboard, but we always were there as any parent would be.

(Funny that Larry says he thinks of me as a son. Years later, I got invited to this medical conference by two different companies. I registered through both and gave Larry one of my old IDs so he could use the second registration. When he signed in, the woman at the desk said, "Oh, I think you already signed in actually." He said, "I get this all the time. There's two Dr. Soloways." I guess she thought he was my dad or my brother!)

Anyway, at the VA, my motivation pushed me to bend the rules a bit—all in the hopes of helping more people, of course. Many students were "practicing" on the veterans at that time. So many patients were enrolled in clinical trials—nothing to the level of the Tuskegee airmen, but disturbing nonetheless. Nearly all of them were made to be guinea pigs as students worked on them unsupervised. What I did, while not exactly on the level, still helped them in the long run.

The Philly VA is where I taught myself how to do lumbar facet injections (much to the chagrin of my professor, the famous H. Ralph Schumacher Jr., as Ralph didn't believe they worked). Lumbar facet injections are touted by David Borenstein, the author of *Low Back Pain*—one of the Bibles of back pain in the United States. I used all the veterans as my own guinea pigs, and I just literally wheeled people down for injections at night by myself. I just started doing injections on anybody who had arthritic back pain. I would go around, and these people would stay in the hospital for weeks and months, and they all told me that because of the injections, they were better.

Some of these patients would practically live there for months. Someone would be admitted for something as minor as a sprained ankle, and they'd stay there *for a year*. They'd go home over the weekend with a weekend pass and come back with their family on Sunday for lunch and dinner. That's the real VA.

People get admitted and treat it as a hotel, when in fact, the buildings probably should be made into some sort of a veterans club similar to the Union League Club, the Elks Club, or the Harvard Club. The VA certainly isn't providing excellent medical care. Across the nation, the VA buildings all look the same, and the care is all at the same sad level.

There's no such thing as "VA doctors." There are military doctors who work at Walter Reed, and these are typically admirals or generals who stayed in the military after medical school. At the VA, though, the permanent staff are all researchers who will see five people here or there. Meanwhile, the VA is really run by the students and the trainees and the residents. It's these low-level employees who make the decisions, almost always at the expense of the patient.

This just proves that there is no such thing as free care—even if you have to wait for days and months to get it in the socialized medical system failing our country. Yet, just as there are people who want to believe in Frosty the Snowman and the Tooth Fairy, there are people who believe that all doctors are trained the same and have the same knowledge. They want to believe what the government tells them: that the VA is equal to, or even better than, the wider healthcare system. In fact, it's inferior. Up until recently, though, veterans couldn't even leave the VA if they wanted to. (Some were allowed to go private on "fee basis" if they were too far from a VA.) Meanwhile, the government was busy negotiating to get the cheapest—not the most effective—drugs.

It kills me, this so-called government rate that they get. If I buy a drug for five hundred dollars, at the VA they can buy the same drug for two hundred and fifty bucks because they get 50 percent off, which is also known as the government rate. I have no idea why I can't buy it at the government rate. (Mexico and Canada must get our government rate as well; the laugh is always on us.) I do know, however, that if I were able to buy the drug at the same price the government paid, I would be able to charge less, make more, and help more people. You should know by now, however, that that is not what our healthcare system is about. Giving people access to healthcare does not mean giving them access to quality healthcare.

Should we even be giving all veterans free access to healthcare, though, regardless of the quality of that care? If you ask me, not everyone deserves it.

In America, we have geniuses who make bombs, and we have regular people who shoot guns. This will never change. There are fifty thousand people in this country who are very smart and are protecting everyone, and then there are two million rank and file who are used as pawns. You can't dispute this.

The fifty thousand elite are on the level of Secretary of State or four-star generals, CIA, FBI, USSS, people who went to West Point, Annapolis, people who want to be career military because they realize the benefit of being in the American elite. (Like the Communist Party, the upper echelons of American society are a closed class in a capitalist system.)

They know that being a military lifer means they'll be taken care of for life in a decent way. They'll never be billionaires (at least not by being in the military), but they can get book deals, TV shows, podcasts, speaking engagements, and other things to help them rise to the ultimate levels of power. Some even ascend to the presidency.

Those West Point and Annapolis grads are the pedigree and the minority. Sadly, the volunteer army does not necessarily reach that pedigree. You know, it's not like 1950, when there was a draft and everybody went proudly. (Even Willie Mays and Ted Williams went!)

Today, since we don't have a draft, everybody who goes into the military is going in by choice. If you're going in by choice, you picked that job and that's your career. So, why are you entitled to a healthcare plan different from the rest of the government employees? We should not treat a soldier any differently from how we treat a TSA worker.

Say a guy joins the army at age eighteen and serves twenty years. He'll be thirty-eight, with a life expectancy of about forty years after that. He should not be entitled to forty years of government healthcare and government pension, until he dies. He should get twenty years: one for each year he served.

I'll say it again: Veterans should not be treated differently from any other government worker—or any worker at all, for that matter. They should not be homogenized out in their own healthcare system. Veterans should be using the same system as regular people, and regular people should be using the same system as veterans. If we're a heterogeneous society, we should act like one.

There's a simple solution to this mess: You bite your tongue, you shut the VA, and you let the VA employees go to work at other important jobs, such as making medicine and keeping the supply lines in the US and out of China. As for the buildings, the VA hospitals are owned by the government, so the government can keep them, sell them, or lease them out. They could use them as pool halls, swimming pools, or rec centers for the local community. They could be sanitariums in the case of a pandemic.

As soon as they're out of the VA, veterans should be awarded a Medicare card, which would ensure that veterans have access to healthcare and their medications. Again, I don't necessarily agree with giving this access to *everyone*. I have a difficult time understanding why someone who serves four years should get benefits for life or, why minor hearing loss sets you up to receive a lifetime of disability pay.

Of course, these are only my opinions; I have no skin in the game, since I don't work in the VA any longer. I merely want to see the medical system function and work for *all* Americans. It's not an impossible feat.

CHAPTER 8
BECOMING THE PATIENT

Sometime around Father's Day 2018, I was attending an event related to the President's Council on Fitness and Health, when suddenly, I fell to the floor with incredible pain. I begged for someone to call me an ambulance. I thought I had a kidney stone, or testicular torsion. It was the worst pain I had ever had.

I'm rushed to the hospital in an ambulance, but I get no special attention. After a while lying around, I finally saw an ER doctor who was probably as old as my kids and as smart as the fish that I had when I was a child. (It was a Kissing Gourami named Charlie.) He says, "We'll do a CAT scan." We do the CAT scan, and he says, "You have a kidney stone."

I said, "Doc, why do you think I have a kidney stone?"

He said, "Well you know, when you get older, you get kidney stones."

I knew he was clueless. "You know," I said, "I don't really see it that way. You know that I'm a doctor, right?"

"Right."

"You know that I'm a presidential appointee, right?"

"Right."

"So you know that I'm not just some schlub," I continued. "I want to be given more appropriate treatment."

The kid was just looking at me with this blank stare. Finally, I said, "You know what? I'm going to leave. Why don't you give me something for the pain, for just a day or two, and I'll go see my urologist when I get home. He's a friend, and I'll have him take a look at the stone."

He says, "Well, you know, I don't want to give you narcotics or anything."

"No," I said, "I don't know. But if you're not going to give me a narcotics prescription, don't even look at me. This is just a waste of my time."

So, I left with a little Tylenol and Motrin, gritted my teeth for a few hours, and called my urologist from the train back to Jersey. I said, "Look, you gotta do me a favor. I'll go straight to your surgery center. I have a kidney stone, and I'd like you to get it out." I went to him and that's what happened. The stone was out, and the pain was over, but the mystery of what caused it—as far as I was concerned—was not.

I brought the original CAT scan from the hospital to a buddy who's a radiologist. He immediately said, "Steve, did you know you have a mass in the pancreas?" (I knew the ER doctor in DC was a moron.)

"Uh, no," I responded. "I don't. Is it that bad?"

He said, "I think you should get it checked out."

I didn't even know what he was talking about. All of a sudden, I was the patient; I wasn't the doctor.

It dawned on me: "Shit. This could be pancreatic cancer."

I called this guy I know, and I said, "I need you to give me a pancreatic biopsy."

He's like, "Steve, what's going on?"

I filled him in, and he goes, "No problem. I'll do it right now."

Within hours, I had a pancreatic biopsy. When I woke up, two gentlemen were standing in front of me: the pathologist and the surgeon.

My friend says, "Steve, I got good news."

I'm like, "So tell me the good news!"

He goes, "Steve, you have a pancreatic neuroendocrine tumor."

I said, "Is it cancerous?"

He says, "Yeah."

"Um, that's what Steve Jobs died of. What's the good news?!" (In fact, Steve Jobs and I were diagnosed with the exact same type of tumor, of the same size, at the same age. Too bad he didn't see Frank Spitz.)

"It could have been adenocarcinoma."

Then, the pathologist left, and another man came in and introduced himself to me: Dr. Frank Spitz, the elite doc for docs who ended up saving my life. He said, "I specialize in internal organ cancers. If you're comfortable with me, when would you like to have your cancer removed?"

I said, "Right now."

Well, it was late, and the nurses had gone home, so he told me that he'd see me the next day.

He says, "Why don't you go home and get some clothes. You're going to be here for a week or two. Come back in the morning, and we'll take care of it."

I checked in the next morning, and after hanging around a bit I had the surgery around four p.m. Keep in mind, I told the anesthesiologist that I'm very athletic, and my pulse when I sleep is forty beats per minute. My respiratory rate is between five and ten. I explained that at that point in the year, I had already swum five hundred miles in my Masters Swim program and I had ridden my Peloton bike more than one thousand miles. Just a few years earlier, I had run in the Philadelphia Marathon. My vitals look different from those of the average person.

Twenty-four hours post-op, I took a walk at the advice of my surgeon. I got back to the bed, and Debra Richards, my CEO, and Chip, her husband, were there visiting. She watched me get into the bed, and I had light conversation with them. Then I started talking to myself, and I fell asleep. Suddenly, all the bells started going off because my pulse hit forty, which signaled an alert for the nurse. (It was forty-one all the time prior.)

Debra explains, "This nurse walks in right past us, totally ignoring what we were saying (Nurse, he just went for a walk and got in bed, nothing has changed, everyone knows he is fit and has slow pulse and respirations. In fact, I mentioned to my husband that doc's heart is so slow, and he is peaceful even after his walk . . .), and hit him with Narcan." The nurse was told I was sleeping and never tried to wake me!!

You may have heard of Narcan. Due to a heroin epidemic in this country, all police and most skilled service employees seem to carry Narcan. If they see somebody having a drug overdose or lying in the street nearly dead from a drug overdose, the protocol is to approach the individual, try to arouse them, and give Narcan to reverse the effects of the heroin, if they appear to be having trouble breathing. Narcan, of course, reverses all opiates.

The hospital staff forgot what I'd told them about my resting pulse rate, and when my pulse hit forty, that was some kind of internal trigger that screamed "drug overdose." My pulse wasn't dropping, and my respiratory rate wasn't dropping. Without thinking, the nurse blindly *followed protocol* and hit me with this serious drug. "She didn't even try to get a response from him or anything," Debra says. "She didn't ask us. We could have told her he wasn't on drugs!"

The result? I went through a death experience. I envisioned myself floating through the atmosphere after seeing an explosion of light that resembled the ice in a movie theater advertisement—at the start of the previews. I was in baby booties and a diaper, floating backward through space. I was yelling as loudly as I could, "I died." I was communicating with Debra and Chip through finger and hand motions. I yelled, "Wherever I land, I will see you there."

In the middle of that noise, I shot out of the bed—literally flew out of the bed—landed on the floor, shit on the floor, elbowed the nurse away from me, and screamed repeatedly, "Fuck you! I will only talk to my physician."

So, the psychiatrist was called. This team (six men!) from security (goon squad) was called, for the guy who was twenty-four hours post-op from the second-most major abdominal surgery you can possibly have, because he was hit with Narcan and is screaming, "Fuck you." Apparently, they made it sound like I was a belligerent, violent drug addict. They lost sight of the fact that I was a post-op patient who had had all of the pain reliever in my body removed, which was why I was probably screaming in pain. (*They either over-medicated me, or committed malpractice by inappropriate use of Narcan—private and confidential sources at the medical center admitted that it was malpractice.*)

Meanwhile, psychiatry forced Debra and her husband out of my room—against their will and against my will—and started interrogating them about "my drug habit."

Debra explains, "I told them that Dr. Soloway doesn't do drugs. I've been working with him for more than twenty years, and if anyone would have known, it would have been me! This man comes to work early and leaves late. He doesn't do drugs. Somehow they didn't get it."

It went on and on. Then, they had the nerve to come in and ask *me* about my drug habit.

I think the first thing I said was, "Go fuck yourself. You either overdosed me, or you inappropriately Narcaned me." (*My notes for those fifteen minutes are missing. Can you imagine? Do they work with Hillary?*)

Landing on the floor was responsible for what became a six-month pancreatic ductal leak. After the leak was discovered, they inserted a tube to drain the leak, and that tube perforated my diaphragm. After the perforation of the diaphragm, all of the fluid they were trying to drain didn't all come out. Nine liters of it went into my left lung. That caused what is called a whiteout.

I could feel some squeaking in my chest and complained about it, so they did a chest X-ray. After the X-ray, they immediately took me to some filthy closet-like room, and the chest tube drained about three liters. They thought it was pus, but it ultimately turned out to be lymphatic fluid. Because it only drained three liters, a week later I underwent general anesthesia to have a thoracotomy and decortication, or video-aided thoracoscopic surgery. The thoracotomy cut a nerve in my abdominal region, so I can no longer have a six-pack. The top-left muscle on the six-pack doesn't even exist anymore. (I have the best five-pack.) I can't feel it, and it's not there. Afterward, the lung doctor told me it could be a complication of the procedure, and he was sorry he hadn't warned me.

If I hadn't done the surgery to get the rest of the fluid out, though, I would have been left with a trapped lung, and I would have had a left lung that was unable to function.

The drain that was left in continued draining for six months.

During the original surgery, they removed my spleen. When the spleen is removed, platelet counts often go up dramatically. Mine went up so dramatically that a hematologist was called (at my insistence). She didn't even ask about the pancreatic cancer or discuss it with me at all. The oncology people totally ignored the fact that I had pancreatic cancer, which is actually a good thing, but still very ignorant and unprofessional.

I got antibiotics—which, it turns out, I didn't need (and there were complications from this, too), because the fluid within me that was thought to be an abscess was simply lymphatic fluid from the lymphatic drain that had been caused when I fell on the floor. (I suggested getting the fluid LDH, and the level came back at 12,000 U/L. There were no cells and no organisms. This is classic chylous fluid from the leak the Narcan *inadvertantly triggered.*)

I had that drain for six months, thinking it was infected, and all the antibiotics gave me a reaction called balanitis. I had to use such a high dose of steroids for the balanitis that I suffered irreversible damage. While I was in the hospital, I developed clots from the IV in my left arm, which led to a prolonged course of anticoagulation.

I am sorry I left out some of the most important details of being a patient. The room was so dirty I had to call administration in the hospital on multiple occasions to have housekeeping—only to be given dirty looks as they actually had to do the jobs. My sheets were so dirty after beds were changed. I refused to sit on the bed and made the people doing beds give me another set of sheets. My shower was broken, and I was forced in my broken-down health to sit on the floor in a filthy shower just to try and wash my hair. The water pressure was so low I had to lean my head against the wall to wet my hair. I pointed out, week in and week out, coffee or other disgusting stains that were on the wall under the desk when I was admitted and remained when I left. Considering the complaints I made to the administration, I am sure they would just label me as a nuisance.

Ladies and gentlemen, this is the real medical system. It only works if you don't need it. I will also share that the hospital itself was so filthy. I was wheeled on a gurney to have X-rays done, past the mounds of garbage piled up in the basement of the hospital. (See photo insert.) If you do not believe me, the pictures are real. I found out that in fact some of my own patients complained to the Board of Health about this same hospital, which was threatened with being shut down. I was so shocked they did not take the threats seriously and had still never fixed the appalling, disgusting, filthy, uninhabitable conditions and what is to be the state's best medical center. Again, bogged down with protocol, the filth was so stuck to the floor the janitor and team used paint equipment or paint removal equipment to actually scrape in my hospital room. The air conditioner controls were in the next room, and I was either freezing or sweating to death and had no control over the temperature, and when asking the staff for help, I was always given a yes, and nothing ever occurred to help or satisfy my problems or complaints. To this day, I continually receive letters in the mail asking for compliments of the health center. Sadly, those who do not know the system probably think they had a great experience because they made it home alive.

Meanwhile, remember that kidney stone? Way back when I had that removed, I diagnosed myself with hyperparathyroidism—something that the clueless ER doc totally missed. After recovering from my cancer surgery and all of the aftereffects, I underwent yet another surgery (exploration of the four parathyroids) to remove the overactive parathyroid gland. Moral of the story: that kidney stone did not happen randomly. I had another condition, and that was missed just like they missed the cancer.

I failed to mention an importance mishap. Two years prior to the discovery of pancreatic cancer, I went to a gastroenterologist and complained of acid reflux. I had an upper endoscopy and was told I had erosive esophagitis. It was explained to me that, because I am a doctor, I got it from being under too much stress. I have no typical risk factors. The main risk factors are smoking or alcohol. Nothing further was done. I also failed to mention that my cancer was producing the hormone gastrin, which was overloading my stomach with acid, thus causing all the erosions that would have led eventually to esophageal cancer. Just another attack of bad medicine!

My longtime friend Kurt Henry was witness to the calamity. As a fellow doctor, he had the same opinion of the whole debacle that I did:

I'd rather be Steve's friend than be his doctor, but I got this physician on the phone for at least an hour. I said, "Here are my concerns. You need to get your shit together. Steve should not be treated with subquality care. You should raise the bar."

As far as I could tell, they had a bunch of fricking foreign doctors who didn't know their ass from a hole in the ground. You can't fool me or Steve, because we've been through this already. We know who these doctors are, and they're poorly trained. They treat patients very poorly.

I said, "I know Steve can be very tough, and he has earned that! I know that. However, he's a great doctor, and if you guys don't get your act together, you're going to kill him. If he lives, there's going to be a lawsuit because my friend is not benefiting from good care."

I mean come on, you do an abscess drain and you puncture the diaphragm and you give the guy a chylothorax. Are you kidding me? It was so hard to watch. Steve called me the weekend before his second surgery, which was done because he had such severe complications. He even sent me the pictures after with his tubes coming out of his chest. Steve didn't eat for four days, he was petrified they were going to kill him, he lost 42 pounds.

He called me and said, "I'm calling because I want you to know you're a true friend, but I may not be around on Monday. This could be it." That's how bad it was. I've seen him exaggerate, *but this, I knew it was true. Steve does not lie.*

The guy was literally dying, and it was because of the healthcare system and how bad the care was.

You'd better believe I want to sue, but nobody will take the case. Three, four law firms said that to have a winning lawsuit, you have to have causation. This truth is to take on such a large case a law firm would have had to lay out close to $1 million and the risk-benefit ratio was not worth the risk. Why bother helping somebody on principle, or do what's just? Easy answer if no money, no principle. Even though malpractice was confidentially admitted already, because the hospital did an investigation, the lawyers say that they can't prove beyond a shadow of a doubt that the Narcan can be linked to the pancreatic ductal leak.

It kept me in the hospital for six months, and even knowing the system inside and out, I couldn't prevent it from happening to me.

According to Debra Richards, "It was a scary time, but Doctor Soloway is a fighter. He pulled himself through it and came back better than ever. He is swimming, biking, and working like a dog."

My story proves that adherence to protocol is far more dangerous than occasional lack of thought. Why would the nurse think to administer the Narcan? It's not like my pulse or respiratory rate was dropping. Everyone knew that my rates were my normal levels. When the bell went off, she acted like a family pet that didn't know how to think. I've even known some family pets to be smarter than that particular woman.

In today's world, nurses—and, for that matter, hospitalists—do not know the patients. As I have explained, your family doctor does not come to the hospital anymore and does not tell you all the nuances of each patient. You are just another number for the hospital. The hospital has bought out the old-school nurse and family doctor and hired people to come in for shift work to do the job cheaper. You get what you pay for. The shift-work mentality clearly fails our system, and this is a great example.

First, the nurse should have known that *Narcan shouldn't be administered unless you try to awaken the patient first.* We know this nurse was incompetent or poorly trained. Second, had the nurse had the thought of giving Narcan, she should have wondered, "How could this patient be walking around the halls with no problems whatsoever just moments ago, yet somehow be overdosing on drugs?" Again, this shows very poor communication between staff and very poor knowledge of what medications the patient has received. Not to mention, if she knew anything at all about me, or checked on me, she'd know that I was a venerable medical professional who had no history of any kind of drug use. It was all a total mess. In the very critical forty-eight hours post-operative, this is when we need our most skilled, most experienced people, not neophytes. It was yet another failure of the system.

The failures of our medical system are not hypothetical. This shit is for real, and it's forever. When I say that our current medical system ruins lives and hurts people, as I know firsthand, changing the system is not about the money for me. (Money is the one thing that can buy you a little more freedom than the next guy, but I'm happy with my life.) It's about the people who put their lives in our hands.

Honestly, the best advice I could give to anyone about our medical system is to try to stay out of it. Ironically, my high-school yearbook quote was, "He who lives medically lives miserably." That's what I have done my whole life, and especially in the years after my cancer. I have to stay healthy for myself, for my patients, my parents, my staff and best friends, and, most of all, for my children. This is what my son, Jake, learned from watching me go through my cancer battle:

> My dad almost lost his life with his cancer, and that whole situation made me completely reevaluate my life. I don't know what I would do without my dad. He is totally one of a kind. I get to see a side of him that his patients probably don't see.
>
> He was always super into Corvettes and still is. When my sister and I were really young, we would go for a drive in his Corvette with the two of us in the passenger seat, and he would blast the B-52's or some old band. We would always call those our "boom boom songs."
>
> On family night, we all would wear matching boxers that we'd call our "uniform." We'd all pile into my dad's bed and watch a movie, usually an older movie like he would watch growing up. He loves *Fast Times at Ridgemont High* and *Stripes*, for example. He will be quoting them in his grave.

He was always my baseball coach and coached every team I was ever on. Throughout my entire childhood, if I ever said, "Dad, let's do this," we did it.

Every summer for nine years I shadowed my dad at his work. I would wear a coat and stand next to him in the room and observe what he did with patients. I was only about twelve, eleven years old, and I was thinking even then that I don't know how he does it.

I've seen some very crazy stuff. We had a guy walk in who was really skinny, and he was wearing a face mask like with the whole COVID-19 outbreak. He looked really, really ill; you just knew something was wrong. When we got into the room, he had warts all over his arms and his legs. It turned out that he knew he had tuberculosis and didn't want to share that with anyone until later. It's super transmittable, so we were all freaked out.

There's always something wild going on over there. Aside from the waiting time, everyone always has the biggest smile on their face when they leave. I love the way my dad talks to patients; it's not how normal doctors talk with patients. That's what makes him unique. He adapts to each person's pace, personality, and knowledge level really well, so they can get a great conversation flowing, get to know each other, and feel that bond with their doctor. That's really important.

I don't get that experience from my own doctors! He's a very special guy. He's a very mentally strong person, and he has very clear and simple beliefs in the sense of being a good person and living a good life. That's all I can strive for.

Living a good life is actually very easy, if you follow my recommendations. First of all, it is important to check in with your doctor every year. Get baseline age-appropriate testing, whether it's cancer screening or simply an EKG or liver and kidney testing. Calcium and Vitamin D testing are very important, because there is a tremendous number of people who have hyperparathyroidism and never find out until they have a kidney stone or osteoporosis, and the coronary damage from the calcifications may be too late for repair. Men over fifty should probably all have their prostate and testosterone checked as a baseline, since men drop their hormone levels just like women drop theirs with age. If your hormone levels are too low, you are going to feel weak and lethargic. Your urologist can handle this problem, find out the reason (making sure it's not a brain tumor), and get your levels back to normal so that you can feel young again.

Beyond that, it is imperative that we all adhere to healthy eating habits and a robust program of exercise. For most adult Americans, it's not even clear what that means. As children, we were indestructible. As teenagers, we were somewhat indestructible. Why? Well for one, Mom usually put three meals a day on the table and forced us to eat. I imagine the typical household—at least where I grew up—sat down for three meals. We had eggs or cereal with toast or bacon for breakfast and had a tuna fish sandwich for lunch with some potato chips, milk or soda, maybe some salad. At dinner, we had either chicken, pork chops, steak, or fish on a rotating basis, with a potato and a vegetable—typically a green vegetable, like peas, green beans, or spinach. There was a variety of foods. Desserts were thrown in once in a while, of course. People were not avoiding sugars decades ago. However, desserts were usually restricted to after dinner, and limited to one portion per person.

Regarding physical activity, all kids used to play outside, probably for an hour or two at minimum, seven days a week. With this way of life, most teenagers were healthy, strong, and at least thought to be indestructible. Well, what changes?

At some point in life, perhaps at age thirty-five, forty, forty-five, fifty, fifty-five, sixty, people become immersed in their own family or in their own career. If they cannot afford to hire a chef to serve up the same three meals a day that Mom used to provide, they end up eating quick and easy food. They load up on carbohydrates and sugars—not protein and vegetables. Their exercise routine goes from several hours minimum seven days per week to none. We are then left with an overweight, out-of-shape, disease-ridden society.

What can we do about this? We can pack our lunch. We can prepare our meals. We can order out less often. We can tell the restaurant to use no salt or less sugar. We can drink our coffee with skim milk. We can avoid sweeteners. We can avoid bread products other than bread that is made with sprouted grains rather than flour.

In fact, there are so many types of flour, we don't need to stick to just wheat flour. Wheat flour is most commonly used, as it has the most iron and the most nutrients of all the flours available. That said, it doesn't taste as good as sorghum, almond, or coconut flour, and it may not have as many nutrients as quinoa flour. It certainly has more carbohydrates than chickpea flour. These are examples of other flours that could be added into the mix. (For those who are concerned, going gluten-free is useless unless you have celiac disease or non-celiac gluten sensitivity.)

What kind of diet should you strive for? Generally, we want a good combination of fats and proteins with minimal carbohydrates, which could be eaten in the morning. A healthy day should start with nut butter or yogurt—plain, of course, five grams of sugars or less. For the nut butter, try walnut butter, pecan butter with cinnamon, crunchy almond butter, crunchy or raw cashew butter.

Cashew butter tastes like some kind of mix between marshmallow and vanilla. If you don't believe me, go find your local brand or search for an online distributor and try it. Tell them I sent you. When you have a big mouthful, it shuts down your appetite and you get healthy protein and good fat, the fat that cleans out your blood vessels.

After your morning snack—and morning workout—have a meal that consists of mostly eggs and vegetables. Don't worry about eating the yolk unless you are eating more than three eggs a day. (You don't want to overdo the eggs, because you can get albumin poisoning.) The yolk may have cholesterol, but it has valuable nutrients, including chromium, which revs up your metabolism. You can enjoy meat or cheese with your eggs, but I would avoid adding unnecessary carbohydrates or refined sugars into the mix. One good choice is huevos rancheros, which gets you a nice mix of eggs, beans, and avocado. The high fat content of avocado suppresses the appetite.

For snacks, I suggest you have a nice piece of fruit: perhaps a nice ripe apple that you picked off of a tree, berries, or pineapple.

Then, for lunch I recommend lean meats such as turkey or chicken, with sliced tomatoes, avocados, onions, mushrooms, and whatever other vegetables you enjoy. If you can avoid bread completely, you can eliminate unnecessary processed carbohydrates, which turn to sugar and make you insulin-resistant. Good bread alternatives include portabella mushrooms or beefsteak tomatoes. If you absolutely cannot give your bread up, then I suggest you use Ezekiel bread. Found in the frozen food section, Ezekiel bread is not made with flour at all, but with sprouted grains. This is a much healthier choice than regular bread for lunch.

For dinner, I would suggest perhaps an alternating schedule of fish, chicken, and steak. If you're a vegetarian or a vegan, you will have to get your source of protein from plant-based products or soy, but this is achievable. A lot of people like to eat kale and other green vegetables. If you enjoy the taste, this is a great way to get protein.

Some of us meat lovers have a hard time consuming enough edamame to fill up one's protein requirement. Still, I am not a fan of protein supplements, although they are widely used. I am not trying to insinuate they are dangerous, but I don't want my kidneys to see a tremendous load of protein. As we get older, there are really only one or two ways to protect our kidneys—other than making sure we are not diabetic or hypertensive. We do need to keep the blood pressure as low as possible, and we do need to avoid big loads of proteins to the kidneys. If a protein load to the kidneys is too much, the kidneys shut down, causing a condition called rhabdomyolysis. This is a very serious life-threatening dangerous condition, and furthermore, it is common. I cannot tell you how many hundreds of cases I have seen throughout my career, starting the first week of my internal medicine residency more than thirty years ago.

Other than that, you probably get the general idea. We want to keep our bodies away from bad fat. We want our good fats to come from nuts and fruits such as the nuts and fruits that I mentioned. We don't need to worry much about the sugar content of berries, because the fiber negates the carbohydrate effect. You will not get a spike in your sugar.

One of my favorite fruits is jumbo Medjool dates. These are from the Jordan Valley or from the California desert. Dates are interesting. They are loaded in carbohydrates, but have such a high fiber content that if eaten one at a time, they do not have a high glycemic index. On the other hand, they do have a high glycemic load, hence you need to watch how many you eat. If this is your only sweet product for the day, then indulge a little bit more.

Don't beat yourself up if your diet isn't perfect. No one's is. I personally have a chocolate addiction. Every day, I find myself nibbling on Hershey's Kisses. I figure it's better than eating whole Hershey bars all day long, but this is not my professional medical opinion. My staff could tell you, I probably have a dozen Hershey's Kisses every day. No exception. If I really want to eat healthy, I'll get the Hershey's Kisses with nuts in them.

Beyond your daily diet, staying hydrated is key, as well. My personal choice for hydration is water; your personal choice for hydration should also be water. Every now and again, I will have a Pepsi to satisfy my sweet tooth, but soda has nothing to do with hydration. When you pick up a soda, you are drinking a can of sugar.

Obviously, no one should be drinking a can of sugar. Starting at about age forty, many of us are predisposed to insulin resistance, also known as Type 2 diabetes. If you want to avoid Type 2 diabetes, you need to avoid sugar. The late great Muhammad Ali once stated that white sugar is poison, and he is correct.

Take a look at the people that you went to high school with. (If you need to go log into Facebook, I'll wait.) Take a look at them now. Most of them wouldn't even fit into pants six sizes larger than what they wore in high school. Why? 1. No exercise. 2. Too much consumption of unnecessary carbohydrates and white sugar. That probably includes beer.

It is reasonable, rational, and healthy to have a glass of beer or wine perhaps once a day, but twelve-packs don't really feature into the equation. If you happen to have two glasses of wine, make it red. Red wine is closely derived from the grape, which means all the healthy nutrients of the fruit will be found in the wine.

That doesn't mean you should plan a day-drinking marathon just yet. Whatever your sassy yoga tank might say, wine is not a substitute for sweat. No matter how genetically gifted you may be, fitness should be a part of your life for your entire life.

While the current mantra is to get children active in sports—and I think that is a wonderful idea—the best approach to creating a healthy society would be to ensure that every person over forty is involved in exercise. I believe it is very important for adults to partake in swimming, running, biking, rowing activities that could be done alone—forever, barring any injuries. It is not enough to be involved in a weekend basketball game, or a summer softball league, either.

For daycare, nursery school, kindergarten, grade school, junior high school and high school, even through college, part of the curriculum should include a class on general physical fitness. Not everyone is interested in team sports. Moreover, while team sports are a wonderful way of bonding, making close friends, and learning teamwork, in the game of life you need to be adept at a sport that you can do on your own. That includes running, rowing, cross-country skiing, cycling, or swimming, which is my personal favorite. Those five activities do not require a partner or a team and provide a groundwork for strength and cardiovascular fitness.

Another often-overlooked activity for muscle tone, strengthening, and hypertrophy would be yoga. Yoga is amazing. If you haven't tried it, I suggest that you do. The injury level is incredibly low. Speaking of which, I'm not a fan of recreational football, hockey, or martial arts. I never met somebody in one of those sports who didn't have serious injuries, and some of the injuries are so serious that people die. There is no reason that your passion or quest for fitness should lead to serious injuries. (I have a black belt in Goju-Ryu karate, however. I used to routinely take down a sparring partner who weighed at least one hundred pounds more than I did.)

Our society is way too focused on professional sports. They play a role in entertainment, just like Broadway and Hollywood, but it's unbelievable how sixteen Sundays go by and fifty thousand people are pumping down the Budweiser, potato chips, Doritos, Pepsi, and Twinkies so fast that they don't even know what country they're in when the game is over. This is all part of the problem. They'd all be much better off going for a hike or a long bike ride.

Whichever form of exercise you choose, you should be doing it five to ten hours per week—preferably seven hours or more, if your schedule permits. Ninety minutes on alternating days could be better for those over fifty or sixty.

Overall, you really need to build regular exercise into your life. Still, I would recommend that everyone take a rest day once in a while. Your body is a machine. If you overuse the machine, skip tune-ups, and don't warm up properly, you will wind up six feet deep. Spikes in blood pressure and spikes in pulse lead to stroke, atrial fibrillation, and other medical conditions that are fatal. Plus, the body does need time to recover and allow broken-down muscle to heal.

Another fitness strategy could be lifting weights—never heavy, because this will probably raise your blood pressure and will tear your labrum of the shoulders and likely the hips. Sorry, no exceptions. If you are new to lifting, have someone advise you on your form, or you could get hurt. With proper form, lifting weights two or three days a week on alternating days—focusing on different body parts—could be sufficient. The other four or five days a week, you should schedule in at least one hour of intense cardiovascular exercise.

I prefer zone training, aerobic, lactate threshold, anerobic. You target different levels of heart rate and/or different levels of intensity for varying periods of time with varying periods of rest on a consistent basis for an hour. This is wonderful for heart and lung health. This kind of exercise fills your

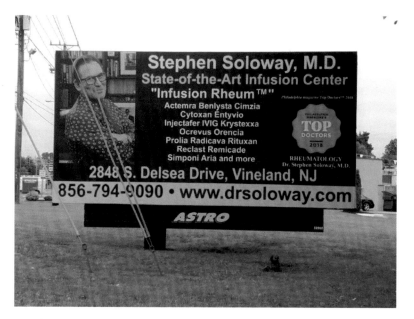

We don't need to advertise. I like the cool billboards, and cool shirts!

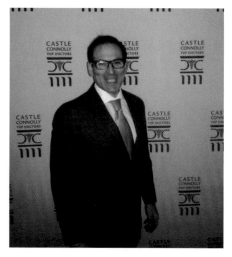

Castle Connolly—Top Doctor (top smile).
(*photo courtesy of author*)

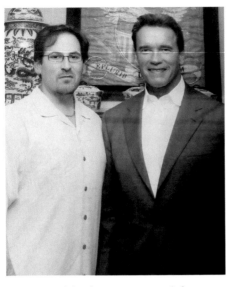

With Arnold Schwarzenegger (*photo courtesy of author*)

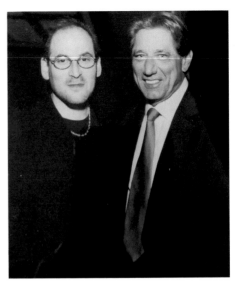

With Joe Namath (*photo courtesy of author*)

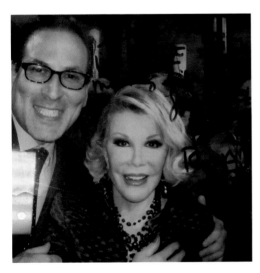

With Joan Rivers (*photo courtesy of author*)

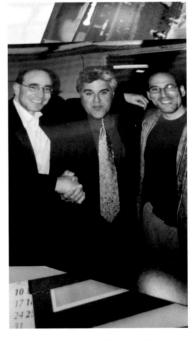

With Jay Leno and David Weksel (*photo courtesy of author*)

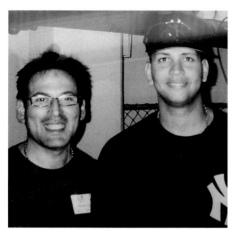

With Alex Rodriguez (*photo courtesy of author*)

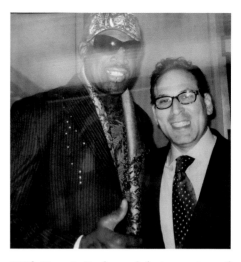

With Dennis Rodman (*photo courtesy of author*)

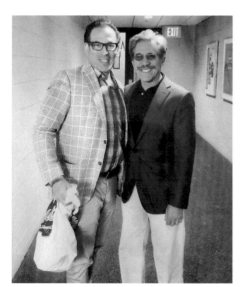

With Gerardo Rivera (*photo courtesy of author*)

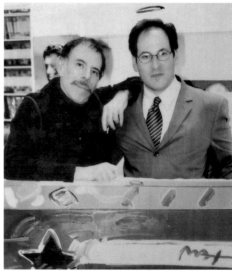

With Peter Max (He seems to think I'm an angel.) (*photo courtesy of author*)

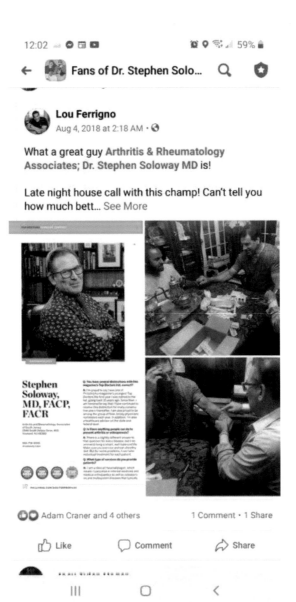

Treating the (Incredible Hulk) Lou Ferrigno

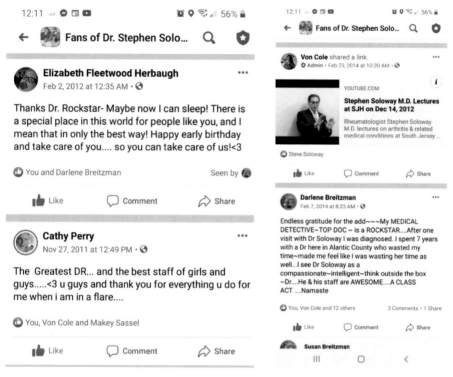

"Fans of Dr. Soloway"—a private Facebook room

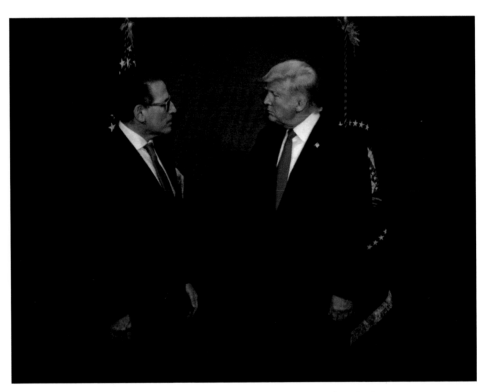

Great conversation, lets speak more soon. (*photo courtesy of author*)

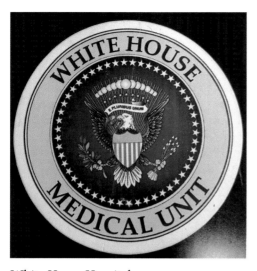

White House Hospital

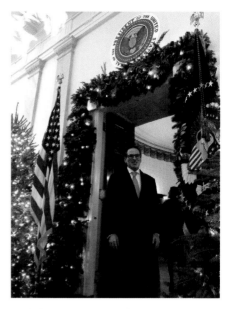

Holiday gathering (*photo courtesy of author*)

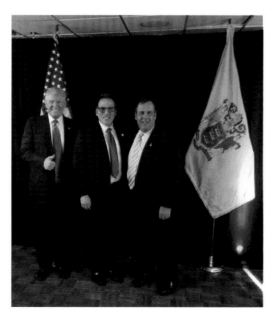

With President Trump and former New Jersey Governor Chris Christie (*photo courtesy of author*)

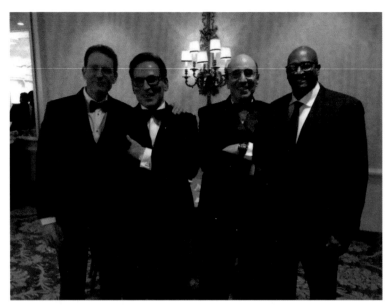

BFFs (left to right): Robert Feferman, "Icon of Dallas," endocrinologist, art collector; David Weksel, businessman and polyglot holder of numerous patents and master's degrees, chess champ, arm wrestling champ, philatelist; Kurt Henry, retired Navy captain, critical care physician, cofounder of DK Star Productions. (*photo courtesy of author*)

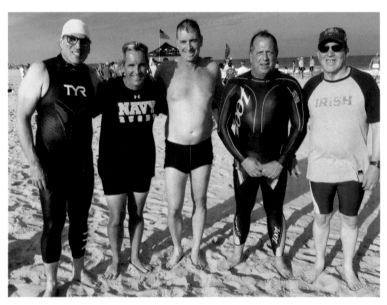

My comrades in fitness, at the Sea Isle Mile Race; (left to right) Steve Soloway (me), Rich Montgomery (president of PTC), Shawn Cassidy (Naval officer, and routinely beats me in 100 freestyle), Mario Valore (youngest D1 athletic coach in history, at age 14, fastest age group backstroke in the world, and outstanding coach), Bill Fleming, the most humble and honest political person around, a standout in NCAA swimming at Notre Dame, even before goggles! This great group keeps me fit day in and day out! (Sorry Erin Callegari Mackey and Liz Barnes Schmidt weren't at the event.) (*photo courtesy of author*)

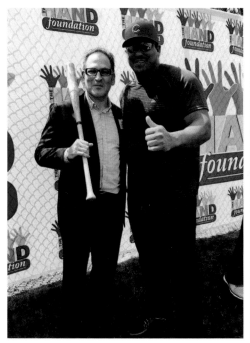

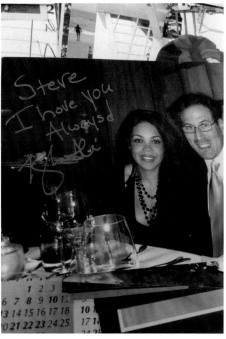

Supporting the Hand Foundation with Carlos Zambrano (retired Major League pitching ACE). (*photo courtesy of author*)

With Khaliah Ali (daughter of the Greatest). She is great as well! (*photo courtesy of author*)

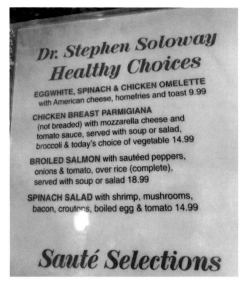

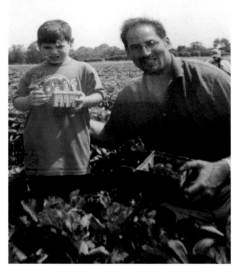

Malaga diner featuring healthy Soloway food choices.

Strawberry picking with my son.

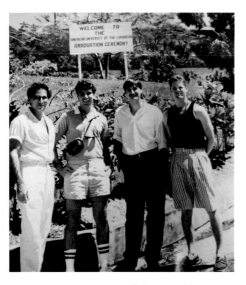

American University of the Caribbean
Graduation Ceremony—1988

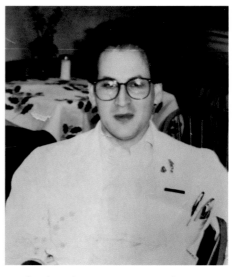

Medical student 1985/6—London

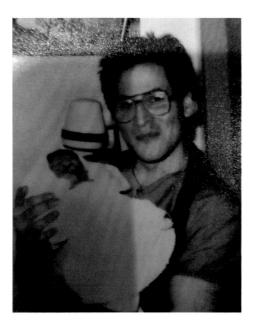

First baby I delivered circa 1986. (She and
I remain friends today.)

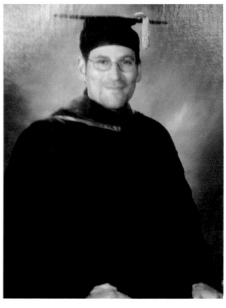

Induction—Fellow of the American
College of Physicians (FACP)

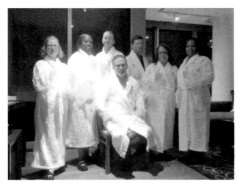

Staff slumber party weekend at the Setai Hotel (Miami Beach). Those depicted above, I don't have enough kind words for you. THANK YOU ALL.

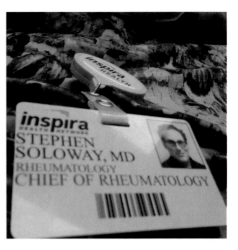

Current hospital ID

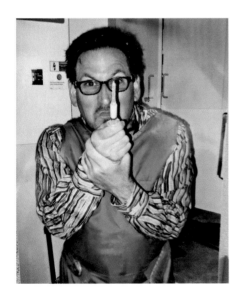

Injection Day. I'm more scared than you!

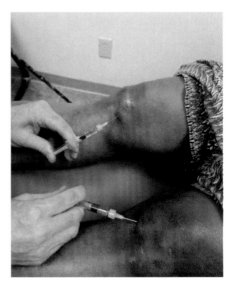

Double shot. Your doctor cannot do this.

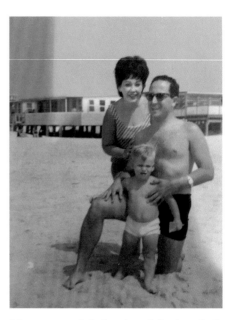

Great-grandparents (namesake).
Sad, the Jews don't often meet their
great-grandparents, as we are not
customarily named after the living.
(Sam never met me.)

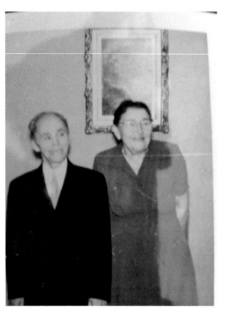

My mom and dad enjoyed the beach. I
don't know how much I liked it from
the look on my face.

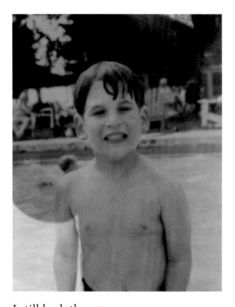

I still look the same.

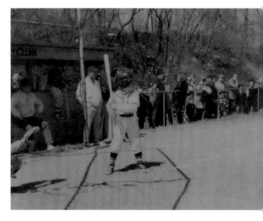

Little League, circa 1971. (It was the
all-star game, I see my Dad and Grandpa
"Tata" along the fence. I homered over the
centerfield fence.)

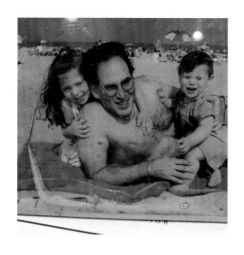

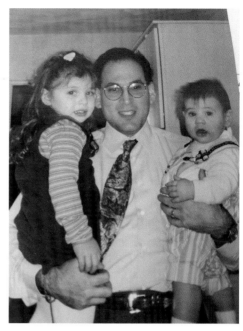

With my little people—Alyx and Jake.

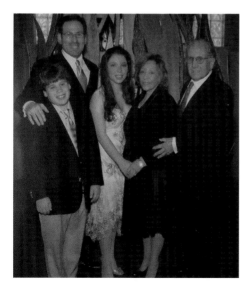

My parents and kids play dress-up on occasions together. (I insist—no one opposes.)

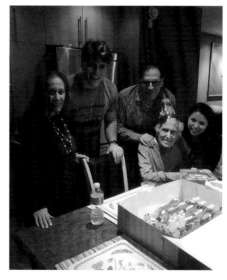

My parents and kids celebrate all.

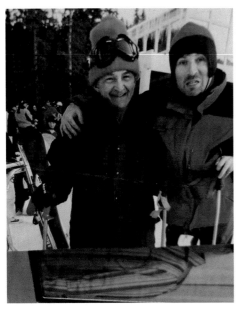

Skiing Santa Fe with Uncle Martin.

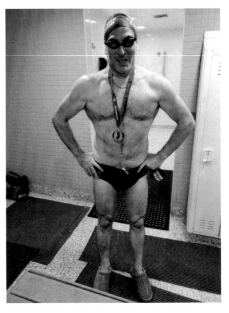

Gold Medal (I really am the best—maybe for my age, maybe not, but I trained like a maniac.)

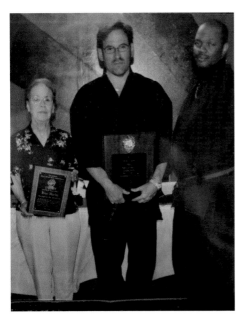

Black Belt Ceremony. You really don't want to be in the way of my front kick. (I'm very passive.)

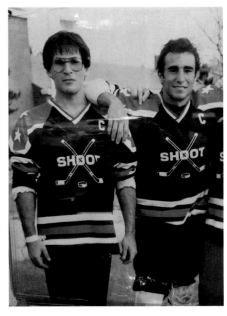

Dave and I—captains of the hockey team. (Who else would be captain—only the best.)

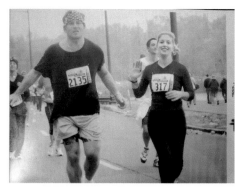

Ran the Philadelphia marathon with AR to keep her company. No one told me to train for this. I stopped to eat chocolate at mile 21. (My headband courtesy of Aunt Lucille.)

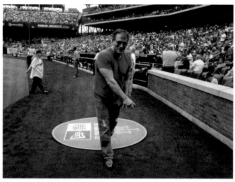

Honored to throw out the first pitch at Subway Series. (Mets vs. Yankees)

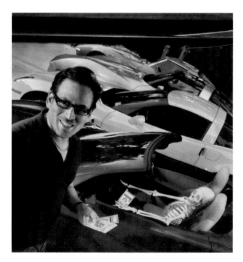

I enjoy fast cars.

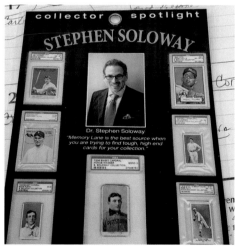

I am the quintessential Collector. I was the king of baseball cards!

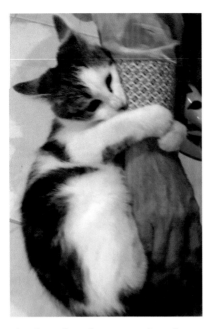

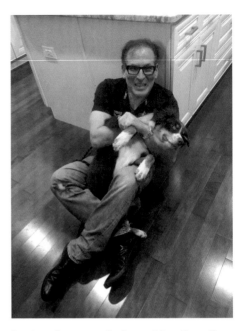

This kitty found in my parking lot, captured my heart immediately, and I never let her go.

I enjoy the pets of others. Meet Leo. I'm his godfather, and we like to wrestle. He is six months old and loves to bite me. My goddaughter Justine keeps him entertained.

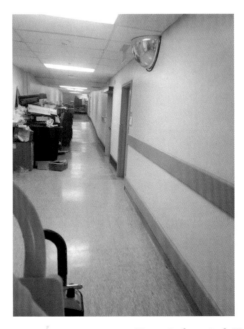

Photo from my gurney on way to X-ray in hospital. You can't make this stuff up. And please try not to be a patient. It's an awful experience. Remember we are "practicing" medicine at your expense—here at my expense. (*see page 140*)

brain with blood (which is a good thing). It keeps your blood vessels patent and keeps you living longer.

If the American people were to adopt this plan, plus the restriction of sugar and white flour, the average life expectancy would probably rise to one hundred very quickly.

Interestingly enough, the reason life expectancy has gone down recently is related more to shootings (Chicago, Portland, etc.) and drug overdoses than to one's health. Occasionally, our most healthy people are killing one another, and that is affecting the numbers. More than likely, life expectancy varies by zip code. Those who live in violent neighborhoods probably have life expectancies of fifty-five years old, while those who are born and raised in places like Beverly Hills or high-rent districts where people are following advice like mine are living into their nineties.

Personally, I'm aiming even higher than that. I believe in the power of routine and following my daily regimen. I just love the bike, either outdoors or with Peloton. I used to run, but after about fifteen ankle sprains, I have no stability of the ankle. After the first quarter mile, I essentially get foot drop and I get paralysis. Instead, the bike is great for cardio, and I'm also a US Masters swimmer. I've been swimming seriously for the last six years, and I swam 150 miles this year so far. Now at time of the writing and summer outdoor swimming, I'm at about 210 miles. (I was stymied by the pandemic shutting the pools.) I was eighth in my age group in the country—now about twenty-third. Prepandemic, I found out I was seventy-second out of about nineteen hundred people, across all ages and both sexes. My coach, Mario Valori, was an Olympic swimmer, and by now I can hang with him during workouts. Don't believe me? Ask Mario!

> Steve has a level of drive and focus that is extremely rare. I gave him a few tweaks on his form when we first started working together, and it's transformed him. Today, his stroke rate is equivalent to that of a professional swimmer.

He motivates *me* to get up early and get into the pool. I don't know how he does it. He works all day, and then he's up at 4:00 a.m. for our workouts. I put the workout for the day by the side of the pool, and he just puts his head down and does it. He's like a machine.

I'm excited to see how far he can go as a Masters swimmer. With his focus and willingness to take direction, the possibilities are endless.

Exercise—whether in the pool or on my Peloton—is a vital part of my day. If I didn't have a routine, I think I would sit in bed all day long. That's where it seems like the rest of the people in this country are going. Don't be one of them.

Before concluding this chapter, I almost forgot to share my experience of being bedridden for three weeks with COVID-19. On a Friday afternoon, my entire staff became ill. Of course, I happened to be the oldest among them and had the most serious illness. I went home not realizing what I was afflicted with and spent five days and nights in bed with fevers of 105 for four hours at a time, and with arthritic joint pain, muscle weakness, fatigue, and extreme shortness of breath. I refused to go to the hospital, as protocol would have had me be on a ventilator—and the odds of living would have been very slim. I roughed it at home by medicating with large doses of prednisone and full anticoagulation and hydration from drinks provided by my daughter. It took between ten and fifteen days before I felt human again, but within four weeks, I was back at work and swimming on a regular basis, as if I never missed a beat. Fortunately, my staff all recovered as well, and any physician friends that I have also recovered very well. Sadly, one of my drivers whom I used for personal car trips passed away after several months dealing with the virus while in the hospital. These facts should never be forgotten. I suffered very badly during that. Fortunately, I am not one of the dead.

CHAPTER 9
BIG GOVERNMENT IS BAD GOVERNMENT

You can't be for big government, big taxes, and big bureaucracy,
and expect personal success!
—Steve Soloway

The US government prefers its citizens be sheep, lulled into submission and ignorance by a never-ending stream of Netflix, Hulu, and Amazon Prime. Archie Bunker termed the TV the idiot box, since, in his words, "idiots watched it." I'm a huge Bunker fan regardless. He was oh so spot on! Uncle Martin was of the same opinion that "watching TV makes you into an idiot." To this day, I concur. There's no thought involved with tuning in and turning off. You don't learn anything by binge-watching, and it's a waste of time. It's for mindless, useless people who waste their lives and just get by milking the system. These people have no desire to learn or see the world. They have no desire to improve in any way, shape, or form. All they want to do is eat Twinkies, fuck, make too many kids, or sit at home on the couch.

A TV is just a big computer screen, and the Internet is even worse of a mental sedative. Morons can fall down Internet rabbit holes for days at a time. It's certainly addictive. I've heard of people who come to work late because they got sucked into someone's Instagram story. They spend the workday fiddling around on Facebook, and they earn a paycheck without putting in any effort at all. What a waste! You can't become self-sufficient playing games of Candy Crush. It's just outrageous. Meanwhile, these people are laughing all the way to the bank on the backs of people actually working hard.

Of course, the computer was a great advance that jump-started our society and put us into a whole new echelon of innovation. Even as I type, the IBM supercomputer is working on seventy-seven million known products that might be able to fight off pandemics. Still, look at all the negative things that computers have brought us. Look at all the computer viruses, all the identity theft, the millions of dollars that have been transferred illegally. There are even hackers that steal the titles for people's homes online. Somebody could probably tap in and launch nuclear missiles if they really wanted to.

Computers have cut my productivity in half, merely by adding to my workload. I have to go back to my computer after every patient and tell the computer what I did, rather than just quickly dictating it on the fly. If you want to keep records in a computer to save space, then great, but it's gone too far. (Oh, the government: Medicare, they insist.)

There's nothing tangible left, because everything's in some "cloud." We don't even produce anything tangible anymore, it seems, except for robots that are going to take away more jobs. Frankly, the robots are smarter and more polite than most people. We're slowly being replaced.

Precisely how the government likes it, though. Our freedom and our free thinking are threats. For example, it continually amazes me that the NRA has been able to keep America bearing arms, but at the same time, we're not allowed to buy the same quality arms as the government. Did anyone ever stop to think about that? Our people's militia, at least according to James Madison, was supposed to be able to overthrow the government, if needed. Our army of Glocks would be useless against the government's tanks, drones, and missiles. We the people have power on a microlevel, but it's all about who has the ultimate despotic power, and the answer is big government. That's all that matters to the people at the top. (This does not apply to any one individual; this is how the system has been ever since Woodrow

Wilson gave FDR the idea for the Bad New Deal. Now some want a bad green deal.)

In fact, the whole premise that this is a participatory democracy is a total farce. With every vote we make, we're buying our own demise. The very concept of campaigning and fundraising is such a massive conflict of interest. Doctors can't go out to dinner with drug company reps, but politicians can steal billions of dollars from hardworking people? "Donate to my cause! Donate to my campaign!" Are you kidding me? People keep buying into a broken system, though, money gets you to the front of the line, and they don't know any better.

The last thing that the politicians should be doing is begging the American public for money, when they're wasting what they already have. I really resent that somewhere between 20 and 25 percent of the GDP is spent directly on the three branches of government. This is not even the rank and file, but the three branches themselves. It's such an endowment, and it's going to waste.

Most people don't realize it, but the federal government—including the executive, the legislative, and the judicial branches of the government collectively—is spending about a trillion dollars a year on itself. This is the same as the Medicare budget, plus or minus 10 percent and the military budget, plus or minus 10 percent.

Where should we start cutting back? Paradoxically, it would be my recommendation that in the future, presidents, Supreme Court justices, Cabinet members, and Congress members all be paid a high salary. The president, for example, would earn a salary upward of ten billion dollars per year. The normal tax rate of 37 percent would apply, and then the president would be responsible for using the rest of that money to pay for his or her own vacations, travel, and security. A president's leisure activities should not be considered a legitimate business expense, and the taxpayer should not be paying for this.

A higher salary would make presidents responsible for paying for their own preferred lifestyle, while the American taxpayer could depend on a set budget for each administration. This would allow people beyond the millionaire and billionaire elites of our country to realistically consider politics as a career. President Trump is a great example of one of the first citizen-politicians we've had for a very long time. Kudos to him. (Although, if you don't speak English well, and you don't believe in Judeo-Christian values, you shouldn't be allowed to run for public office. Being a citizen is not good enough. Plus, nobody under the age of forty-five or fifty should be president. No one has matured enough until that age.)

You're probably wondering: With sky-high salaries, wouldn't elected officials be more useless than ever before? Wouldn't they be constantly campaigning to hold onto their seats and their paychecks? It's likely. That's why I believe we need draconian term limits. Six years for all, and never two terms. Justices can stay for life: they carry the values over generations, and they hopefully maintain their values with time, like a navy suit.

You should not be allowed to have a lifelong career as a politician, period. Allowing that has made the government a kind of shadow communist party of rich elites running a supposedly free country full of sheep. Some of these elites are worse than Putin. See: Ted Kennedy, not quite a pillar of what Harvard is supposed to represent. He clearly showed that liberal elites can get away with murder.

Yes, there's some balance of power in that the states, counties, and cities are allowed to govern themselves to some extent. If the government decides to come in with martial law, it's over. People will experience the full reality of the system that we've created.

Presidents should only have one term, although it should be six years, enough time to fill your promises but never a distraction looking for a second term. A president needs to have enough time to make good on his or her campaign promises. They shouldn't spend time strategizing and campaigning for the next election.

Until then, just know the government will crush you whenever they get the chance. To quote George Carlin, "They own you." They have unlimited time and resources; you don't, because you have to work for a living instead of sucking money off of everyone else.

Anyone who is self-employed—from your local small business owner to Jeff Bezos and Mark Zuckerberg—knows that the government will drop the hammer on anyone who gets too powerful or too successful for their own good. It's stupid, there's nothing the government can do better than the private sector. Literally nothing. Everyone in the government works on fixed income and fixed time frames. There is no sense of urgency. In the private sector, you have highly motivated individuals who are high achievers. To the government, the successes of the private sector are mind-boggling, they can't comprehend it. They think people must be bending the rules and come running immediately when they smell success.

That includes me. Once I started earning more, something got triggered in the halls of government, from DC all the way to New Jersey. I was added to some kind of list, and they decided it was time to make my life a living hell.

For example, I do many facet blocks per hour—very prolific and organized. Facet blocks are a minimally invasive type of joint injection. All of a sudden, I got a notification: Your volume is too high, and we suspect foul play. I was audited; they found nothing wrong. Case closed, right? Wrong. They audited me more, and I'm sure they're not done.

There should be rules around auditing. If you find me to be acting criminally, then shut me down. If you audit me three years in a row and don't come up with anything, then get the fuck out of my life forever.

It's not just the feds that are on my case. In 2005, I started small joint MRIs in-office for the convenience of patients, and I had outside radiologists read them, so there could be no user bias. From 2005 until December 31, 2008, everything was great. Unbeknownst to me, on January 1, 2009, the laws to operate MRI machines supposedly changed from that day forward. (Or did they? The Department of Environmental Protection Radiation Protection Element and the medical board were on different rules—one had no clue what the other did.) New Jersey required MRI machines to be state licensed, whereas prior to this date, there was no need to be licensed. They did have a grandfather clause to protect some practices: if you had been in practice before 1991, you were exempt. They probably knew that I started my practice in 1992, so I was not covered. This was portrayed to me by counsel. Frankly, I said, "just settle asap so I can sleep at night." The BME (Board of Medical Examiners) asked me to stop using the MRI since they couldn't verify the images to be clear visually. Meanwhile, the NJDEP Radiation Protection Element allowed for "unlicensed MRI by private offices." Truthfully, I never would have made an agreement that still lingers, as my records prove the BME and the NJDEP Radiation Protection Element were not on the same page, and when the board asked me to stop as above, they themselves had no idea whether I was allegedly not in compliance with some ordinance or another. Finally, I found data that it is legal for any doctor to have an MRI in their own office.

Other rheumatologists were doing MRIs at the time, but I was a big gun. However, I couldn't't be grandfathered in (so I was told by counsel). This, in spite of the fact that I was credentialed with every insurance company to do small joint MRIs (I won the X-ray contest at UPenn two years in a row; no one ever did that) and that it was a benefit to my patients—saving them from going to the hospital and paying an additional charge. I saved the system millions, by avoiding hospital fees and patient copays. Millions of dollars is how the issue made its way to the state government.

They (DOBI) fined me $250,000 and prohibited me from doing MRIs. (I had already stopped when asked, and to this day I never saw the law that prohibited using the machine.) The whole thing was sent to DOBI, the New Jersey Department of Banking and Insurance. Under the guidance of my attorney, and in fairness, not knowing the future ramifications and not being explained how this system really worked retrospectively, I would never have signed an agreement, and frankly, I believe I will be able to get the signed agreements overturned, as there is overwhelming evidence that there was nothing wrong that I have done.

Eleven years later, though, they are still harassing me and want to officially reprimand me. With a public reprimand already issued through DOBI, it feels like this is getting redundant. It's adding salt on the wound (or piling on, as they say in football) by going after my medical license, which has nothing to do with this.

What a waste of taxpayer money. The sad thing is, it was all because I was making money and helping my patients. Even though overall, the system was saving money, they only saw that Steve Soloway was making too much money. They're so short-sighted. Nobody in the government is ever looking at all the good things I do. They're just saying, "Well, he makes too much money, and we're going to fuck him."

Despite the fact that I sit on the BME and am the Chairman of the South Jersey Preliminary Evaluation Committee (largely due to my cool shirts), they won't let it go. None of it is about due process. With the Board, the decisions are made before the process begins.

In New Jersey, the hierarchy of the Board can be jaded. I take the Board seriously and have tried making suggestions about how reprimands and other punishments should be doled out, but my thoughts are viewed differently from those of the majority.

We have people selling blank prescriptions, and they get suspended for something stupid like three months or six months. They go to California, and they start practicing all over again like it's no big deal. Others get much more draconian sentencing for minimal offenses, just because they're on someone's shit list. Once, I was so agog at the obvious enmity of the board to one subject, I said, "Why is this physician even getting a trial, when it's clear the decision has already been made against him?"

One of my fellow Board members told me, "Well, he is entitled to a trial. He is *not* necessarily entitled to win."

In most cases, a "win" isn't even the end of the battle, though. At least with the State Medical Board of New Jersey, a "win" means the physician is required to go to an administrative law judge for review (if there is a judgement against the practitioner). If the judge disagrees with the Board's decision, his or her ruling is not final; the Board gets to disagree and act like it is a superior court, rather than a bunch of nonlegal scholars fecklessly doing what they choose.

They choose whom to go after. They cut deals and turn a blind eye when those who are recused *unrecuse* themselves for the purpose of passing a vote. It's despicable, to say the least. The rules change as the wind blows, except the same person makes all the rules and the wind never blows the same way. Nobody stands up to them because most doctors are too busy trying to make a living. Not even the Manhattan plastic surgeons would be considered truly wealthy in today's economy. The corruption continues, year after year. Again, the patients are the ones who suffer for it.

Congress isn't much different. In the case of the federal government, it's the American people who are the unwitting victims. Imposing term limits would help clean the mess a little bit. In politics, too much experience guarantees that you're corrupt. That reminds me of one of the most important lessons I've ever learned: If a politician asks you for a favor, say yes. They might not ever pay you back for it, but if you say *no*, you better believe they'll seek revenge—someday, somehow.

Another way to drain the swamp (our current Congress) would be to institute limits on congressional pensions. Under the current system, members of Congress are eligible for a pension at age sixty-two after just five years of service. That is insane. I firmly believe that you should put a year in, and get a year out. If you go to Congress and you worked there for four years, your pension's four years—not more.

Congresspeople also get incredible health insurance better than that of any working person. You need to explain to me why these people earn $193,000 max per year and get a health insurance plan worth roughly two million dollars. Nobody else could afford something like this; how can they? They're not self-employed. They didn't earn anything. All they're doing is following the well-worn path of the career politicians—the gravy train.

Why should politicians work for four years, six years, or eight years and have free health insurance and pensions for the rest of their lives? It's ridiculous, particularly since they are supposed to be public servants—and go back to their own careers after service. Heroes like Willie Mays and Ted Williams sacrificed their prime earning years in the military, and they didn't get that kind of deal when they got back. Congress shouldn't get it, either.

If the politicians know they're not going to get lifetime benefits, we're going to get rid of a lot of the slackers. For example, a guy like Chuck Schumer. I can't say anything good about him, except that he should retire. If not, maybe they could actually fire him. I won't hold my breath for an impeachment trial for him because the system's not fair. It's corrupt, and by now we all know that. My disdain for Schumer stems from a fundraiser I attended on his behalf. I proposed a medical legal question. His response, "I have many doctor friends at Harvard," completely ignored little ole me. He is the scum from outer space.

Is there any aspect of our current government that I *do* actually agree with? Believe it or not, I think we should all pay our taxes. The tax rates as they stand are very commensurate with what we get out of it. (I should say, they are reasonable in certain ways, and unreasonable in others.) I am happy to pay my taxes, and all other people who earn an honest living should pay taxes, too. Why? The answer is simple. The federal government is here to keep the peace. It's because of them I do not need an armed guard to walk down the street (maybe I will if the left takes over), and I do not need tanks mobilized so I can drive to work. If I lived in a socialist or communist country and I needed to go to work, I would be paying more than my 80 or 90 percent tax bill for it (just as Bernie Sanders would like it), and I would require personal security, as well—not to mention the cost of a helicopter to get me to my office, like they do in crime-ridden Rio de Janeiro.

I do *not*, however, believe in taxes at the state level. If I ever become governor of New Jersey, the very first thing I would do would be to cut the state tax from 10 percent to nothing. (However, I *would* want a line item as to where every dime from the casinos and the turnpike goes and would legalize marijuana and add those taxes.)

If you look around the country, this seems like an obvious decision. Florida and Texas have very robust economies and no state taxes. Meanwhile,

California and New Jersey are taxing people to death. Everyone leaves those states. It's the billionaires who are leaving, and that hurts the state in the long run. The states will go broke. The only people left are civil service workers who just follow orders and do what they're told to do. Too much taxation trends to socialism, and socialism kills off the entrepreneurs by taking away their motivation for innovation. If you have no entrepreneurs, you can't create jobs; and if you can't create jobs, you create even more of a financial burden on society. It's a vicious cycle.

Speaking of jobs, though, it's not just the entrepreneurs that we need. The worker bees at McDonald's and Walmart help our economy run, too, and we should make it easier for them to make a living wage. I don't mean we should raise the minimum wage for everyone. Instead, I would propose a two-tier system.

There needs to be a separation, and people need to get off their high horse and accept it. First, say you're a fifty-year-old man who is a good person and holds a job at McDonald's. You have a wife and two or three children, and you and your wife both have minimum-wage jobs. The minimum wage for those people should probably be fifteen bucks an hour or more. Let's call that the "provider" wage.

Now, if you're under twenty-three and you're working at McDonald's too, night and weekends while you're in school, that should be called a "dependent" minimum wage. Those people should get seven or eight bucks an hour. I'm sorry, if you're a high school student scooping ice cream, you shouldn't make more than that. Any more money in your pocket is going to get you in trouble. You're not paying your rent with that money or buying baby food. You're not taking that money to the stockbroker. You're buying drugs or another pair of sneakers.

Starting with that dependent wage, you could graduate up into the provider wage and build a life that way. Say you worked for twenty-five or thirty-five years (which is how long people in this country *should* work to keep our economy functioning). Your retirement age, or the age where you start taking benefits and/or pension, should not be a fixed number. In addition, you should receive a number of years of benefits that is equal to the number of years you worked.

Keying Social Security to age sixty-two, Medicare to age sixty-five, and other benefits to a particular age is stupid in every possible way. For example, if I start working for the FBI when I am nineteen, I'll be subject to forced retirement at fifty-seven and a half. You're telling me I have to go find a part-time job until I turn sixty-two? No. You need to put me on Social Security when I retire at fifty-seven because you, the government, forced me to retire. I put in thirty-nine years of work; I deserve thirty-nine years of pension, which would take me up until the age of ninety-six.

On the other end of the spectrum, if you're a healthy, active eighty-year-old running your own company, why should the government send you a monthly check? Some people at that age don't even *want* to accept it. They certainly don't want to retire. Let them keep paying into the system and give them a bigger monthly check when they're finally ready to retire. It just makes sense.

If I ran the government, I would immediately implement the notion that to get a year's pension, you have to do a year's work. That includes Congress, the president, the enlisted man, the postal man, the fire department man, the policeman, any man or any woman, period. You put in twenty years of work, you get twenty years of pension. That's it.

Most people will have to work forty years to be covered by Social Security in their golden years. The days of people dying in their sixties and seventies are over (unless we all get killed by coronavirus, of course). The only exceptions would be for people who are injured on the job, permanently and truthfully. Say someone shot a policeman. That officer gets free healthcare the rest of his life, and he gets free pension the rest of his life, too—as does his immediate family.

In my case, for example, I graduated medical school in 1988 and started my practice in 1993. If I decide to retire when I'm sixty, I'll have put in thirty-six years. Shouldn't I get to decide it's time for a break then? Why should I keep working for the two extra years? If I want to retire after thirty-six years of work, then my retirement age should be whatever age I am when I've worked thirty-six years. My government benefits have to kick in for the amount of years that I had when I retired. If I think I'm going to live to be a hundred years old, I'll retire when I'm sixty, and I've been working for forty years. I don't want to rely on anybody, and I'm expecting my life expectancy to be a hundred. So, I have three or four more years of work in me. Of course, I'll still work part-time afterward. Who knows, I might even have time to write another book. (To my beloved patients: Don't worry, I have no intention of retiring anytime soon. I love my staff and patients way too much to stop working.)

***

I include here a letter from one of my esteemed colleagues who is fighting the government tooth and nail. Read his rendition below. If the government does not act to eliminate "Surprise Billing," your health care system as we know it will cease to exist. There will be no choices—only socialized medicine. The poor will continue to get bad care. The wealthy will continue to get the best care they can afford. And the middle class will be left with no care.

How We Can Remove the "Surprise" in Healthcare

Dr. Michael H. Brisman

CEO, Neurological Surgery, P.C.

Over the past two years, the issue of surprise medical bills has risen to the forefront of the national healthcare debate. These are bills that patients receive unexpectedly from their physician for care they have received, usually in an emergency. To properly address this critical healthcare issue, two changes must happen.

The first is rhetorical. The term "surprise medical bill" is a misnomer. It was concocted by the health insurance industry—and is continually peddled by its army of lobbyists, bankrolled "experts," and academics for hire—to paint physicians and hospitals as the bad guys. In the real world, there is nothing surprising about these bills. They reflect the normal charges any given surgeon, radiologist, or a host of other physicians routinely bill their patients. The real surprise is that the patient's insurance plan refuses to cover the bill. This debate, therefore, should revolve around the real issue at hand: these bills are actually unpaid insurer bills.

The second change is practical. Unfortunately, with the help of their supporters in Congress, health insurers also have been pushing for a so-called solution to this problem that, unsurprisingly, would be a cash cow for them. The Senate Health, Education, Labor and Pensions (HELP) Committee, the House Energy and Commerce Committee, and the House Ways and Means Committee have all done the industry's bidding. They have offered legislation that lets the government impose price controls and "benchmark" payment rates for physicians. This is the health insurance industry's nirvana. A benchmark payment rate is not only the rate of its choosing, but also an open door for the industry to further drive down payment rates in the future. This would be the final nail in the coffin for independent physician practices across the country. Thankfully, we do not need to socialize our healthcare system with price controls to solve this dilemma.

The best way to eliminate these bills nationwide is for Congress to implement a fair independent dispute resolution (IDR) process. This is a system that allows both sides of the billing dispute (insurance company and physician) to submit all relevant information to a neutral arbitrator for a final decision on the disputed payment. This IDR process is already being used in New York (Out-of-Network Law, 2014) and Texas (Senate Bill 1264, 2020) with great success. If New York and Texas can agree on something, it must be good.

Many patients don't know Congress already has the solution right in front of its face. The answer is H.R. 3502, the "Protecting People From Surprise Medical Bills Act." This bipartisan legislation has been sponsored by Rep. Raul Ruiz (D-Calif.), an emergency physician, and Rep. Phil Roe (R-Tenn.), an OB/GYN. The bill allows physicians and insurers to resolve disputes through negotiation with a fallback to a neutral and fair IDR process. This approach removes patients from the dispute and treats insurance companies and physicians equally. With 110 cosponsors from each side of the aisle, this is our best bet to solve the scourge of these unpaid insurer bills. As President Trump faces an uphill battle in these last few weeks of the campaign, he would be wise to support a fair IDR process, too. That would be a win for him, and, more importantly, patients and our healthcare heroes.

CHAPTER 10
SOLOWAYISMS

I love aphorisms like a fat kid loves cake. (I'd fight mom for the Hostess cupcakes after bedtime.) I use them daily and never the same twice. If tape-recorded, my "Soloway book of aphorisms" would be the best. I should know: when I was twelve, I was that kid.

Yes, I'm a big personality with an even bigger vocabulary, and I've always found apt expressions in colorful turns of phrase. Here are some of my favorites:

If you want it done correct, do it yourself. (I trust you get it!)

Eat to live, don't live to eat. (Eat smart, live longer.)

If it happens once, it's a trend. (Learn from history.)

The devil you know may be better than the devil you don't. (Be careful what you wish for.)

If you don't get what you want, you may deserve better!

Never say never; never say always. (Especially in medicine or exams.)

Stand for something or fall for anything! (Follow your dreams and do not be so gullible.)

Cream rises to the top. (The best will always prevail.)

If you're in Texas and hear hoofbeats, it's probably a horse, not a zebra. (This is a very helpful metaphor in medicine, similar to Occam's Razor. You'll see more common problems than rare diseases, and this is important to understand and use in diagnosing. For those of you who aren't familiar with Occam's Razor, there's always Hickam's Dictum: "A patient can have as many diseases as they damn well please.")

If you're not going forward, you're going backward. (Credit to Uncle Martin, but I've still been using it for thirty years.)

Watch out for number one, and don't step in number two. (I taught Uncle Martin that one.)

Communism is great as long as you're in the party. (See: Chapter Eight.)

Strong moms make strong men. (See: Me.)

The harder I work, the luckier I get. (This is a lesson that I have tried to pass on to my son, Jake.)

Money is power, and power is freedom. (You can buy your way to the front of the line and get access to those with even more power than you. You can set policies and change laws!)

Common sense is not common. (Unfortunately, I know this from experience.)

Stupid is ubiquitous. (This follows from above.)

Nobody's equal. (If we were, this would be a sad and boring world to live in.)

The only thing fair in the world is the bus fare. (Some people don't even get that much.)

If you're not part of the solution, you're the problem. (This is true when it comes to our nation, the healthcare system, and even the minor annoyances of daily life. Quit whining and start working.)

You snooze, you lose. (Don't wait around for your ship to come in. Swim out to it.)

Even the blind squirrel sometimes gets a nut. (Even a total nut sometimes stumbles upon a granule of truth.)

Even a broken clock is right twice a day. (Even our pathetic healthcare system still manages to save lives.)

Diseases don't read textbooks. (For those of you who aren't doctors, any disease can present in any fashion, so as people all look different, diseases all can express differently, too. There is no substitute for hands-on experience.)

You don't treat test results. You treat people. (If I've said it once, I've said it a million times: Don't ever come into my office and tell me, "The blood test said . . ." I'll be the one making the diagnosis, not the test.)

Trust no one. (Except me, of course.)

Look out for yourself, make no deals with the devil. (Success doesn't require sacrificing your ideals.)

I don't need to be the richest person in the world, as long as I have all the money I need. (Is that too much to ask?)

Freedom is expensive. (What price are we willing to pay?)

You can't change a broken system. (When it comes to healthcare, I'm willing to try.)

Visualize success and don't allow anything to stop your desire to get your expected outcome. (That is a playbook for a great life.)

You can't fix stupid. (Self-explanatory.)

Be giving; favors are more valuable than money. Use favors for yourself alone and use them wisely. (Remember that others are keeping track of the favors that you owe them, too.)

Life is a marathon. Planning and training are mandatory. (Don't spend years sitting on the couch and expect to win a prize.)

Don't let losers upset you. You can't avoid them, so plan the trip. (In fact, you should be flattered when idiots aren't a fan.)

Success and power will find you, provided you put your energy and resources into it. (There's enough out there for everyone willing to work for it.)

No one is worth going to prison over. (Nothing is, either.)

It's more gratifying to hit a triple than to be born on third base. (Most of us were born in the dugout anyway.)

Hard work beats talent when talent doesn't work hard. (Dedication plus drive beats them all.)

You haven't achieved any success until you've made a few enemies. (I've told my mother this many time over the years. I suspect after this book, I'll have a few more enemies—and likely more success, too.)

CHAPTER 11

TRUMP

Steve Soloway is a great friend of Donald Trump. I know, as I'm Steve Soloway. Some of his infamous slogans including "Fake News," "Chyna," and "Make America Great Again" make me smile and see his elaborate way of thinking and communicating with all parts of society—a real, down-to-earth guy! He loves a great steak, M&Ms, and Diet Coke, as do I. He has charisma and knows how to bring out the best in people. Yes, I am proud to call President Donald J. Trump a longtime friend. We're a lot alike, Donald and I. In fact, some people have called me "Dr. Trump" over the years. The only difference? I'm neither wealthy nor POTUS. Finally, what the country needs. He is the first TRUE CONSTITUTIONAL CONSERVATIVE IN MY LIFETIME. Adroit at dealing with China, he sees the risks of Chinese aggression, takes all measures to mitigate China threats, and God help us if a rogue, demented, democrat gets in. America may cede.

I have been so enamored with Donald. Over the years, he became a household name in my parents' home. We have gotten to know each other well over the years, as we share common interests. We are go-getters and job creators and hard workers. He has often been a source of both inspiration and advice. I will say, no one knows how to live life like DJT. He gets my vote for *Time* magazine Man of the Century. With huge successes in real estate, golf courses, entertainment, and becoming president, can someone accomplish more? A leader and inspiring.

One of my dearest BFFs, Rob Feferman, has seen my relationship with the president develop over time. He says, "Steve has been friends with Donald for a long time. He sends me pictures of them on the Trump plane and things like that. It's funny, sometimes when I hear Donald talk, I can close my eyes a little and think of Steve. They both enjoy golf!"

How did it all begin? Donald and I first crossed paths shortly after 9/11— which, coincidentally, was right after my disaster of a divorce. I went to New York looking for investment properties, such as easy-to-manage condos in great locations easy to manage, since I run a medical practice. I discovered condo-hotels, or hotel-condominiums (invented in large part by DJT) where I could have my cake and eat it, too. This is one of the most brilliant concepts imaginable. I could use it when I wanted, and the rest of the time the Trump Organization rented it for me. We'd share 50 percent of the profits. It led me to copyright the phrase, "A bond you can sleep in."

I started cherry-picking apartments that were listed at half-price. After 9/11, real estate prices dropped a lot in Manhattan: 1 Central Park West (a.k.a. Trump International Hotel and Condominium) and virtually every other Trump hotel property that existed. I picked up many condos, over time. Before long, Trump sent Jim Petrus (the COO of Trump Hotels) to find out who was buying these apartments. An amazing man and great friend now, Jim found me, brought me in for lunch, and that's when I met Mr. Trump.

When Trump found out what I was doing, he treated me like family. At a condo Board meeting, I got into a verbal argument with somebody on the Board, which almost led to a donnybrook. Trump called me into his office right after. I thought I was getting kicked out, that I'd blown my chance at being close to his greatness. (Of the many, many things that I admire about DJT, his most admirable quality in my eyes is his knowledge and ability to live life to the fullest.) Instead, he told me he liked my loyalty, courage, fortitude, support, and strength.

Mikael Damelincourt is currently the managing director at Trump International Hotel Washington, DC. He and I have enjoyed a close relationship as the Trump empire grew. Mikael explains:

Dr. Soloway and I met in late 2007, when I was one of the executives in Chicago for the Trump condo-hotel concept in Chicago. Dr. Soloway had purchased units.

He's a very bright doctor, but he's also a very bright businessman, and a great human being. He actually helped me a lot. It was new for me to do a condo-hotel concept, and he helped me tremendously to understand—from an owner standpoint—what was important for them. It was just a tremendous help for me to get the project going.

In a condo-type concept, investors like Dr. Soloway buy a unit and then they give it to us, the hotel management company, to run it for them. They can come use it as they wish, and enjoy the services, but then they won't make any revenue. My understanding is that Dr. Soloway owned a number of units at several Trump properties.

He came for the inauguration with his family in 2016. It was an incredible time.

For Dr. Soloway, the inauguration was a really, really special moment. How many times in life do you attend a historic event of such magnitude, after all they only occur every four years. It was an emotional moment for many people, including Dr. Soloway, and being in Washington at that time was a lifelong memory. During the inauguration, I had the opportunity to introduce Dr. Soloway to my family.

People like me are in this business for a reason: we enjoy people. Many of my guests, like Dr. Soloway, have become my friend. Over the years, I've gotten closer to some people more than others, but you end up knowing a lot of people. I spend a lot of time in the bar and all the restaurants at the property, for example. Small groups of people often gather, especially in the evening, and many business relationships are created in that ambiance.

I've also had the opportunity to see him with his children. They're both very bright young kids, and he's proud of them. In watching him over the years, I can tell you that he has been a fantastic father to both of them. You can see the connection that he has with them. Myself, I have young kids. When I see people with adult children who have done very well for themselves, like Dr. Soloway, I hope I can do as good of a job.

I know I mentioned this at the beginning, but I want to reiterate that he is an incredible businessman. I can see that in the way he has invested in the condo-hotel, and the choices he made with his investments. What is perhaps most important, though, is that he is a great friend, and he's a very loyal person. He's been very loyal to me, and he has a big heart. He will do anything for his friends. He has always been 110 percent behind me, behind my coworkers. Working with other property owners, I can tell you that combination is very, very rare to find. He should be commended for that.

Through Mikael, I met a dear friend named Michelle Renee—an image consultant and fellow Trump supporter based in San Francisco.

Beyond his intelligence, Dr. Soloway just had such a great sense of humor and was so off-the-cuff, with a true zest for life.

He told me that he's a patriot and conservative, and we talked about how no one thought this day would come (except Steve said he knew all along). We celebrated our mutual interest: this country, the president winning. Since then, we've kept up a correspondence about all kinds of topics.

You can always get the straight answer from Dr. Soloway. He's very direct, but at the same time he is very choosy about who he speaks to. You don't know who he is unless it's been communicated to you. I like to say that he's like a red onion: They're so different from white onions, or yellow. There are so many more layers. If you cut it, you'll see how dense it is, with so many layers. When I say layers, with someone like Dr. Soloway the information about him unfolds as he allows it to unfold. Still waters run deep. That's his intrigue. You don't get to know someone like Dr. Soloway unless they want you to know them.

Meanwhile, political strategist, policy advisor, and commentator Martha Boneta has been someone I have become privileged to know. She explains:

Steve and I have developed a relationship as people that care about the future of our country. He has a breadth of knowledge far beyond the medical field. His insights into politics, policy, and more are always valuable to me and so many others. I'm blessed to have him as a friend.

My relationship with Mikael and my connections with everyone in the Trump orbit are invaluable and exceptional. My relationship with Trump himself is cherished. Meeting Donald Trump and being acquainted with him for the last eighteen years has been the best thing that ever happened to me. Paradoxically, it's also been the worst thing that ever happened to me—through no fault of his, of course. Let me explain.

Perhaps the most valuable lesson that I learned from Donald Trump is that I learned how to see life through the eyes of a billionaire. That's a blessing and a curse. I'm a very motivated person, but he motivated me even more. I got a glimpse of what it looks like in the levels of society that I had never visited. Don gave me a tour of his private plane and told me that if something happened, they wouldn't't look for him or me first in the wreckage. Instead, he pointed to a priceless Renoir on the wall. That was an instance where I could see how he appreciated accomplishments of greatness, how in tune he was with his surroundings, and how carefully he curated his life to be surrounded by things and people that he enjoyed. (Coincidentally, since Renoir had rheumatoid arthritis, I knew his art immediately.)

Personally, I don't want to go to the moon, but I sure as hell want to see the subway under the White House. I've been in the White House—toured the East Wing and the West Wing and had lunch at the Navy mess hall in the West Wing.

It is all incredible. Yet, these are places that I can't always go to. I can only go if he takes me, and I can only stay for the five minutes we're there. Like I said, it's both a blessing and a curse to know what's possible in this world, but some may be just beyond your reach.

Still, I've done well for myself, too. By the time I was thirty-five, I was wealthy by my family's standards—even though in reality, I wasn't wealthy at all. My mom said to me, "Having money's nice, but having money when you're young is nicer." It's very true.

I've always loved my toys. I'm basically a young kid who never grew up. Over the years, I amassed what was once the world's most impressive collection of baseball cards, known as "The Steve Soloway Collection." I made it into the Professional Sports Authenticator Hall of Fame because my behemoth collection was so revered worldwide. To this day, it is still mentioned on social media as one of the greatest of all time.

I like fast cars, and my favorite has always been Corvettes. I love McLarens, too. I love art, as well. I imagine I have the collector gene: some coins, old paper money, stamps, art, rugs; my favorite artists include Leroy Neiman, Peter Max, Sandy Cohen, Anna Privaloff, Steven Katz, Michael Godard, Tom Ferrera (Willem de Kooning's first assistant), and Dale Chihuly.

I enjoy New York memorabilia and Americana. I have a real mailbox, like from a street corner, in my foyer. I didn't steal it, but somebody knew how bad I wanted one, and he acquired one and refurbished it for me. (Thank you, RV!) In addition, I have a real payphone that works. For the pièce de résistance, I'm looking for a 1965 Bel Air checkered cab. I want a police car from New York from the early seventies. I'm dying to get an old New York subway train car delivered out here. If you know a guy, give me a call.

Perhaps Trump influenced and further inspires my taste for enjoying all that life has to offer. He is a man who knows how to enjoy life. We are both very confident people with formidable but lovable personalities.

I visited him on the set of *The Apprentice*—meeting all the stars and smelling the limelight was fun for me. I do love the burgers in his building that was home to the filming!

Trump appointed me to the President's Council for Sports, Fitness, and Nutrition. It was a great honor, and the most memorable part of it was getting close to Lou. At the first meeting of the PCSFN, I challenged Lou Ferrigno to an arm-wrestling contest, which led to our friendship, and was graced with helping him professionally.

My vision for the council focused on keeping elderly people moving, whereas the council believed that school-age children should be having fitness as part of their everyday routine. Government shouldn't't be raising our children. More money should be invested in keeping the elderly moving so we can keep them out of hospitals.

With the onslaught of COVID-19, many of my colleagues and patients have called for me to join the president's task force, I explained he knows other reputable doctors. Honestly, hydroxychloroquine is routinely used in rheumatology. At the end of the day, when POTUS suggested hydroxychloroquine for COVID, he wasn't wrong for trying, as the drug is safe as water, especially with short-term use. Fake news was rough on him for that and comments regarding bleach and sunlight. Again, fake news distorted his words. He merely said that various things sound interesting. He never suggested anyone drink bleach.

He sure has his hands full dealing with a lot of swamp people, throttlebottoms, and uncooperative sorts. Whether you call it the deep state, or the lifers, sadly they run part of the country, too. The Secret Service and the military industrial complex have a hand in running the country. They have too much power.

As a president, you do have the power of celebrity. Since Trump already was a celebrity to begin with, he has more power and cachet than the usual commander in chief. Being a celebrity has many perks, Air Force One, Marine One, your own hospital, and invites by the most distinguished people living on Earth. He is a man who was born to *be* the spotlight.

I sat at Trump's desk in New York for five minutes during his campaign and was in awe; the people and attention were overwhelming me.

Watching your friend vet vice-presidential candidates and become president of the United States is beyond surreal. No one deserves this platform more than he, and overall, he's done a great job so far. I am especially impressed with lower taxes and repatriation of money.

His first policy that made a lot of sense to me is that you have to be accountable, and you have to work. His second policy that was a winner was to repatriate the money that had been lost overseas. Basically, by lowering corporate taxes, Trump brought Apple back, along with billions of dollars. That was terrific.

The fact that my federal tax bracket went down 2 percent under Trump's new tax plan is great. I can no longer deduct my New Jersey state tax. Many billionaires have left the state for that reason. Now, Congress and the state government say, "Hey, it's not our fault you live in New Jersey." Meanwhile, the state can tax me to death until I just say, "I'm quitting."

Everything he does is a fight with Congress, and he has to wrangle all of the idiots underneath him. He's in a difficult position. He expected other people at *his* level to be as hard-working, principled, and dedicated as himself, and it's very disappointing to find out that nobody is.

It's been unbelievable watching Senator Schumer—who ten years ago was Trump's number one ass-kissing sycophant—turn into one of the most acrimonious pieces of rotted carcass floating around in the swamp that is our Congress. I was at Donald Trump's office years ago when Schumer came calling and was *begging* him for support and campaign money.

It's hard to pick who's in second place when you have such strong candidates to follow Schumer, such as nervous Nancy Pelosi, dummy Dianne

Feinstein, or "The Squad," headed by AOC (Anarchist or Communist?). My vote probably goes to the mawkish and capricious Ms. Pelosi, who has been arousing anger and frustration in the general public by accusing the president of not performing his duties, when she was the one who delayed the Paycheck Protection Program from getting through Congress. What a hypocrite. President Trump perfected the art of the deal; Pelosi and Schumer perfected the art of the canard.

And the mayor of NYC, what a beaut! Hundreds of thousands leaving, crime, graffiti. Destruction of neighborhoods and communities. Some by the idiot himself. Perhaps a tax hike will stop the shooting and looting? If you really are disingenuous enough to defund the police, we should get tax cuts to pay for private security. Remember, mayor, you reap what you sow. Mayor Giuliani is a hall-of-fame mayor, you are in utero.

CHAPTER 12
PANDEMIC

Just this morning, I was forwarded a video clip: Trump issues order to bring troops back to active duty to assist in coronavirus response. It's official: we are in the middle of a third World War. How did this happen?

It's clear to me that the COVID-19 coronavirus was a pathogen produced in China with the intent of killing protesters in Hong Kong. It's since gotten out of control, far beyond anything that they ever imagined. (Although, maybe they *did* hope that it could make its way to the United States all along.)

China was trying to avoid having egg on their face in front of the international community. (Please, let's not have any more photos of tanks facing down protesters like in Tiananmen Square.) They set up the perfect assassination plan with the perfect alibi: we'll make a killer virus that looks like a natural flu epidemic, and then when we get through the outbreak, we'll have the world's sympathy and support. Obviously, it didn't go that way.

All of a sudden, the woman who told people to get masks has disappeared. The scientist who came out of the lab that mutated this virus was killed or died. The world economy has ground to a halt. The whole thing must have taken so much planning; you have to give the Chinese credit. If this were a movie, I'd give it five stars! Best of all, the whole world still believes that it was just bad luck that the outbreak started in the heart of China. The only way that China could have done better is if they moved all of the people from Wuhan into Hong Kong for the experiment.

Don't believe my theory? You will. I'm smarter than the average person, and my intuition is right 100 percent of the time. Why is it so far-fetched to so many? Planes were grounded from Hong Kong to China, but not from

Hong Kong to Europe or the US. How on Earth anyone could blame Donald Trump for this is just beyond me.

The Chinese are far from stupid. They are well-trained soldiers from birth. They are trained communist spies who have infiltrated our infrastructure for the last several decades, sabotaging our government and our most precious secrets. They want to be the ultimate world power, which means destroying America. They're even willing to sacrifice their own people in doing so. (If you get the virus in China, you go missing, or they house you in one of their four hundred comfortable concentration camps, rather than treat you!) Really, they're worse than ISIS. Americans, on the other hand, are not prepared for this.

In times of peace and stability, *Americans are able to maintain the illusion of freedom and liberty*. Now, facing chaos, it is easy to see how thin the line is between prosperity and utter destitution. As society faces more stress, people will default on loans, banks will repossess homes, and the government will repossess properties from the banks. Even if you sell your house, the government will take a cut of that, too. In essence, it is becoming clear: we don't really own *anything*.

Everything is owned by the government, at the end of the day. Some people have their heads in the sand, so this revelation doesn't affect them just yet. Others have been watching their assets dwindle and years of hard work disappear into thin air as the economy crashes. Interestingly, the stock market has done reasonably well, but this does not help the working-class family or the masses. It's clear the writing is on the wall, even now in August 2020.

As I write, we are about 30 percent of the way to a worst-case scenario of "only" 1.0 million deaths. (It would have been a lot more, if not for President Trump's leadership.) The other three hundred million people watching the carnage will have a rude awakening, too. What separates them is only some small unknown differences in their immune systems—a difference that as of now is not scientifically understood. What many people do not understand is the difference between exposure to the virus versus infection from the virus. We all have risk of exposure, and once exposed some are unaware, some go on to die. What is known is that most die from breathing complications. These complications can be overwhelming virus load, blood clots, thromboembolic disease, or cytokine storm. At the time of this book, there is yet neither vaccine nor cure. There are therapies used for each of the above problems, which can shorten one's hospital stay, but nothing more than that. Of the many vaccines being experimented with, the one that I favor is interesting because it targets the viral DNA with memory T cells and it targets the RNA with antibodies. The NIH apparently disagrees with me and did not list that company with the few that got billions of federal dollars. All other vaccines work on RNA only, which means the virus can still be mutated. In my field of rheumatology, we have noted many rheumatic connections to the virus including arthritis and a symmetric pattern similar to rheumatoid and inflammatory muscle disease and weakness and a mimic of lupus involving the lung, to name a few.

Even in rheumatology, I emphasize the importance of the omnipotent internist, Nick DePace, with whom I work closely and have discovered two unusual COVID cases.

I am coauthor with Nicholas DePace et al. on a July 24, 2020, article in the *Journal of Medicine* titled "Unexpected SARS-CoV-2 cardiorespiratory arrest in a myopathy patient undergoing immunosuppressive treatments: A case report." I have a second case report in manuscript form titled "Lupus pneumonitis masquerading as COVID-19 pneumonia."

Beyond the deaths, an unfathomable number of people are about to go bankrupt and/or commit suicide. Many people will lose assets—even the rich. Hard to believe? The average American does not understand that businesses and real estate take money to maintain after you buy them. Many property owners won't be able to pay the property taxes or HOA bills needed to keep what they own, and the billionaire class will swoop in to take more assets from hard-working Americans yet again. The same pillaging is happening already on the stock market, where the ultrarich—even in our Congress!—are scooping up stocks that the less wealthy have been forced to offload. This will linger for a generation, and printing money is not the answer, as the GDP-to-debt ratio can only rise so high before the country is insolvent. We don't want our bonds downgraded again—this would be catastrophic.

The financial disaster will show the very thin line between communism and capitalism. The internal components of the government are already acting like a communist state: seizing goods, businesses, and supply lines, while the others try to make do with the scraps that are left.

The scraps in our country are usually enough for people to believe that they're free. What a delusion. Sure, some people will be getting a couple hundred bucks from the IRS, but it's not worth the greater cost. I personally received a wire transfer from Medicare out of the blue, but after reading the fine print, I send it back. They are preparing to audit anybody who takes the money, within two years. I have to waste my time filling out paperwork just to return money that I didn't't want in the first place. Typical government bureaucracy. If you think the government is really helping Americans with this bailout, think again. The government will always take care of itself first. They send everybody money, and then they tell you in the fine print that if you don't use the money properly, you're going to jail. They will charge you with the False Claims Act, which is a felony. It's a setup.

There's such a total double standard. The government made suggestions, in this case—that people should wear face masks and wash their hands, don't touch their eyes, any time they leave their homes. These suggestions seemed delayed due to leftist politics. Even if it took months, they should have issued every citizen a military-grade mask that could be worn through any chemical or biological attack. If the president has one, so should your grandma. Anyone who's been in the Capitol building knows that there's a cache of hazmat suits for everybody that works in the building, hidden in white crates every dozen yards in a hallway below the building. We don't need full hazmat suits, but the government should have issued gloves, too. (I was calling for it on my Facebook page in January or February.)

We must reopen the country—the schools, first and foremost. Don't tell me it's too expensive; the government just printed four trillion dollars. The left is trying to keep schools closed, business closed, borrow more money, and the Democrats want raise your taxes to pay back that money—ironic, since they have been capricious, starting with the NIH.

Why can't people easily find N95 masks to buy? The government has already taken them all. Homemade masks have helped this problem, but you realize there is no proof that they work the same, better, or worse; however, the NIH had to issue a statement to keep people happy or at least content. Even in times of peace, the government has an unfair advantage when it comes to securing medical supplies. You might not know this, but the government has the ability to unilaterally set the prices that it desires to pay companies for medical supplies. The average doctor or hospital is *not* allowed to negotiate the same price, which is called the "government rate."

It's an incredibly strict mandate. I once negotiated so well that a supplier told me that they must give me rebates, rather than charge me the price we had negotiated. According to my contact, they would be in a lot of trouble if they were found to be selling something to *me* cheaper than they sold it to the government. This is not OK.

It's not OK that the government got a head start on securing masks and other supplies, and the rest of us are supposed to play catch up to get into compliance. Meanwhile, the feds continue seizing the orders that states and hospitals have managed to get on their own, so they can fill the federal stockpile and play politics with who gets the goods.

Constitutionally, the states are supposed to run their own business. When Jared Kushner said that the states should have their own medical supplies, he was right from a true constitutionalist standpoint. Per the Constitution, Congress is really only there to levy taxes. Now, that's all fine and good, except for the fact that nobody has followed those rules for the last one hundred years. The government changes the rules whenever they want, but we're still supposed to follow them blindly. It's absurd.

The real losers are average Americans. The situation is abysmal. The number of unemployed went from three million to twenty-two million to thirty million. It is widely anticipated—and I believe, correct—that unemployment will stay between five and thirteen million or more for at least one year, likely longer. By the numbers, our economy is crippled and, even with government stimulus, will likely remain crippled for a generation, if for no other reason than the fact that all of the money being put out by the government now will lead to hyperinflation and higher taxes later. In reality, the effects of this pandemic will last decades.

Trump was faced with two options. Both choices leave him in a precarious position: have the people to return to work or ask people to stay at home. Of course, it's clear people must return to work. People will remain afraid, and society as we know it will grind to a total halt for years or more. If he follows the advice of the doctors and keeps people out of work, he'll have to accept the fact that society will never be the same again. These are both checkmate situations, at least in his mind, and the end result could be as drastic as a civil war.

We are seeing civil unrest. Has anyone seen Portland, Minneapolis, and Seattle lately, to name a few? With so many officers and first responders becoming ill, or morons suggesting defunding the police, we are already seeing many abandoning their posts. Looking at the example of the USS Theodore Roosevelt, we can see that the military is under great pressure, too. Worse, China is now pushing boundaries in the South China Sea. In the Spring of 2020, the Chinese aircraft carrier Liaoning, and a carrier task force of five other ships, including frigates and destroyers, sailed right past Okinawa. All the recent activity there is a clear show of aggression, which furthers my theory that this virus was no accident. It's imperative that Trump get reelected, so when China inevitably shows aggression to Taiwan, we can stop it. Otherwise, Taiwan is going to be a country of the past.

Will America become a country of the past, too? California Governor Gavin Newsom is calling his constituents a "nation-state" and making moves that are almost tantamount to secession. Can we stop our nation from cracking at the seams? Abraham Lincoln said, "A house divided against itself shall not stand."

It's hard to fight an unpredictable enemy, but the only way to save our country is for the government to start thinking of this situation as our generation's Manhattan Project. This is an all-out attack, the Pearl Harbor of our time. The only appropriate response would be for the president to invoke the War Powers Act and order all pharmaceutical and biotech companies to immediately halt all research and developments to focus 100 percent, twenty-four-seven, on getting a vaccine (at the time of this writing it seems we may be nearing a vaccine within six months). There should be a biologic warfare division sitting down to make sure that we have a vaccine in three months—not coming up with reasons why it has to take a year. Nothing else will solve the crisis. The best chance would be a vaccine that targets the nucleus and the capsule by different mechanisms.

Let's be clear, though: the president should not have to invoke the War Powers Act to get people to pitch in. Why didn't companies already make ventilators—and, for that matter, dialysis machines—here, instead of shipping them in from China? Why aren't US drug companies making the pills we need? You should not have to beg TEVA in Israel to make more Plaquenil because there's a shortage for the people who actually take it (all lupus patients and some rheumatoid arthritis patients). All companies and leaders should be thinking about what they can do to help our nation stand on its own two feet again.

Let's see if these businesses and billionaires will get to work to save our country, and not just for the publicity that every company seems to be chasing right now. From Bill Gates to Elon Musk, everyone's announcing their own donations, their own initiatives. They want the credit for what they're promising, instead of linking up with others to actually solve the problem. The resulting brain trust would be so much more valuable than some CEO throwing a million dollars at it. Big donations for PR are just like throwing cash out the window. It's not really doing anything beneficial for anybody. Perhaps the world's twenty richest should donate twenty billion each anonymously (thereby avoiding selective favors later) and eliminate the virus and defend from all future biologic attacks.

I'm sick of the PR circus where anyone with a TV platform automatically makes themselves an expert and the savior who knows the secret that will end this pandemic. The other day, Bill Gates and Sanjay Gupta were on some CNN show. First of all, Bill Gates essentially spoke as authoritatively as if he were an epidemiologist. Meanwhile, he's a fucking tech giant. Sanjay Gupta, the supposed physician, was sitting there saying, "Oh yeah, that sounds really good. Yeah. That's pretty cool. Yeah. I think I agree with you."

Gupta is the stupidest guy out there. He's a retired neurosurgeon who got a gig on TV and seemingly forgot everything he ever learned. Instead of making himself some kind of news anchor, Gupta belongs saving lives. Instead, he'd rather bask in the spotlight than actually help people. Greed is driving his career decisions.

Regular Americans are greedy, too, but if all of these talking heads and tech kings actually do care about saving lives, it's time to prove it. I'm hereby issuing a challenge to our best and brightest: Get off social media, put your heads together, and let's split this atom. We have to do it, and we have to do it now. There needs to be a real sense of urgency—not just for these business-people, but for all of us. Moreover, a shared project like this might be the only way to truly unite the country at this point.

The next few months are going to be very telling in regard to what being an American truly means. Can people put aside their egos and differences of opinion, and pull up their pants and get to work?

I'll be looking especially closely at our Congress. It's harder than ever today to effect real change at a federal level. The people who are making the big decisions are so well off and utterly disconnected from the real world. They have no sense of urgency, because they are so far removed from the true effects of the pandemic. It's just another partisan argument to them. For example, the Democrats voted against the four-trillion-dollar stimulus, and the stock market fell 5 percent. They stopped the vote because they wanted to push their own agenda instead of saving lives and businesses (Democrats wanted the money for their progressive agenda and figured they would leverage anything to steal taxpayer money, thus delaying needed money for those 30 or 40 million out of work). They don't see or care how their decisions—or lack thereof—are affecting everyone's lives and bank accounts. That's why they decided to take a vacation (Congress should not be allowed recess or even a weekend off if there is a crisis) in the middle of what is potentially the greatest crisis our country has ever known.

Until a true course of action is set, the government should suspend trading on the stock market, except for private individuals who want to liquidate their assets. I don't even know what that would look like, but the volatility only seems to be adding to the general panic and confusion right now.

My fear is that the longer Congress dillydallies, the more companies will go out of business. Those losses could become permanent. Moreover, people need to realize that it's not the loss of jobs that is the biggest threat to our economy right now; it's the loss of job creators. Entrepreneurs and small businesses are supposedly what make America truly great. If they are burned, the future of our economy turns to ash, as well.

We need to act now and put all of our nation's efforts toward finding a vaccine. Notice that I say vaccine and not cure. That's because—sorry to say—there will never be a cure. There's no cure for HIV, and they've been working on that for decades. There's no cure for herpes (nor for cold sores, nor for shingles). There's no cure for the common cold. After all of our lifetimes, there are still no cures for measles, mumps, rubella, polio, rabies, Zika virus, human papillomavirus, or any virus, except for Hepatitis C. Viruses are nasty, tricky, and cunning. The best we can do at this point is to prevent people from getting a full-blown case of COVID-19 at all, with a vaccine.

I believe that China already may have a vaccine, and that they gave it to all of their party leaders and spies a year ago before unleashing the virus on the Hong Kong protestors. Of course, they'll never share it with us because they want us decimated and weak. We have to do this for ourselves, and if they can do it, we can.

First things first: even in the best-case scenario, a vaccine is not going to be available next week. A proper vaccine(s) must successfully complete

Phase 3 clinical trials and hopefully be rolled out soon thereafter. It's going to take some time—at the very least, until the end of this year.

After that, the next step would be to develop a wider treatment with antiviral efficacy. As it stands, we do not have the technology available to fight other viruses that could spill off from COVID-19. What happens when we're hit with COVID-20? We must work to develop a broad penicillin-like drug for viruses. We do not have it today, but we are close enough that a full-court press over the next year or two might lead to a true antiviral that could be effective in a more global sense. We could make sure that we never have to go through a crisis like this again.

If we are able to develop a vaccine or antiviral, we need to make it available to all Americans across the board—not just the military and first responders. Why is it that only people in the military have been vaccinated against anthrax, and the rest of us have not? Anthrax is just one biological agent out of hundreds that we've identified. Smallpox is eradicated because of vaccines. Polio is eradicated in the USA because of vaccines. Anthrax (not a virus) is not eradicated, so the vaccine should be readily available. The COVID-19 virus is just one example of an infinite number of pathogens that can kill people and destroy society. They're swirling around our nation every day. Our vulnerability is just more obvious now.

Every American should be vaccinated. Didn't we learn a lesson from the polio vaccine? It ended a crisis and created one less major headache. We are now seeing the dreadful effects of the coronavirus, and a vaccine looks like the best option. The anti-vaxxers need to give it up and get in line. Lives are at stake. (Of course, they'll all scream about leaving our country if we mandate vaccines. No matter how many people threaten to do that, no one will. They never do. Those threatening to leave for political reasons should surrender their passports immediately and not even come back for a vacation. As much as they may hate whatever it is they hate here, there is no place better. If I am wrong, why have any of the haters not moved permanently to another country—regardless of party affiliation or political beliefs?)

In the meantime, what about hydroxychloroquine, also known as Plaquenil? Originally developed as a malaria drug, Plaquenil has not been used for that purpose for years, due to chloroquine resistance. Today, it is most commonly prescribed for lupus patients. Fox News reporters have made no secret of their belief that this drug could be the coronavirus silver bullet the world has been waiting for. Sorry, but that's total BS. There is no treatment of any kind with proven value at this point. (Remdesivir is shown to reduce hospital stay from fourteen to eleven days.)

Initially, one Plaquenil study from France followed thirty people (which is not enough to call it a real trial anyway). Of the thirty people in France who received the hydroxychloroquine, one went on to die, which is a fatality rate of over 3 percent. That's already more than double the worldwide fatality rate at this time, which hovers between 1 percent and 1.5 percent. Of the rest of the thirty people in the trial, a handful had to be put on a ventilator. Isn't it obvious?

As I have said from Day One, this can't work. If Plaquenil worked, we wouldn't need social distancing. If Plaquenil worked, there wouldn't be one thousand people a day dying. It doesn't work. As of this writing: 180,000 dead, 12,500 nursing home dead, 75,000 presumed dead winter 2020 before COVID testing—that's over 250,000 dead!

You can't treat herpes with penicillin, period. (By the way, there's never been a study on the use of penicillin for herpes, but anyone will tell you it doesn't work.) You can't put out fire with gasoline. I'm sorry, but you don't need trial and error for this one.

The one positive result that hydroxychloroquine seemed to accomplish in the thirty-person French study was that it reduced viral shedding. Viral shedding refers to how quickly a virus can replicate and spread itself within the human body. However, the goal of treatment is not just reducing viral shedding; it is saving lives. The drug cannot do that.

If you *really* wanted to stretch the possibilities, consider that they gave six days of Plaquenil in the study. If you wanted to use your wildest imagination, you could say that if you timed it right and you gave a patient hydroxychloroquine six days in a row when they're shedding the most virus, maybe you could limit the shedding. That's the most you can say about it. What does that even mean? Does limiting the shedding even accomplish anything? Not really. It doesn't lessen the symptoms or really improve the prognosis for patients.

What's more, the Z-Pak that they seem to be recommending that doctors prescribe along with hydroxychloroquine is only good for the pneumonia (most pneumonias have turned out to be viral, in fact) that often follows a COVID-19 infection. It will do absolutely nothing to the virus itself. In sum, this mix is not a cure, it will not save lives, and that's final. If people think it's going to save their life or people claim that it did save their life, it didn't; they would have lived anyway.

In the meantime, what's the harm in them continuing to test that mix? Is it true, like the president said, that we have nothing to lose? In defense of President Trump, the drug *is* universally safe, so those who take it according to direction won't be harmed. In thirty years of prescribing the drug, I've honestly never seen a side effect. However, even aside from the fact that there are idiots out there who fed themselves fish tank cleaner, the answer is that, of course, we have something to lose.

Hydroxychloroquine is safe, if given in the proper dose. In extremely rare circumstances, negative side effects can include retinal toxicity, if the drug is taken for years in high dose. If you go to the eye doctor and follow directions, however, that is reversible. You might see cardiomyopathy, which can lead to heart failure, but that is exceedingly rare and after decades on the drug. I know this firsthand because I have been prescribing Plaquenil to my patients for thirty years.

Lupus patients need this drug to function, and they will be the ones hurt if we continue to waste Plaquenil on COVID-19 cases. (There is scientific data that Plaquenil or hydroxychloroquine reduces lupus flares, lupus renal disease, lupus arthritis, and lupus rashes. Plaquenil even lowers cholesterol.) I've already heard from my local pharmacists that the government is seizing up what's available across the country, in the hopes that it could be a cure.

It's already become harder for lupus patients and other people with autoimmune diseases to get Plaquenil, which will lead to inflammation and flare-ups across the country. In turn, these people will become more vulnerable to contracting the virus. It will be a vicious cycle.

A lack of Plaquenil is going to cause mental health issues for these patients, as well. Just imagine it: if you're on a drug that's kept your chronic disease stable for twenty years and somebody tells you that you just can't have it anymore, of course that's going to make you angry, frustrated, depressed, and anxious. People will get mad, and people do bad things when they're mad. This is all going to lead to higher cortisol levels in that population, which could trigger flares. It's a disaster waiting to happen. The best course of action would be for the president to disavow this idea immediately.

Instead, treating patients with the plasma of previously infected and recovered patients sounds promising. But it needs further testing.

Testing for infection is becoming more available, and that will help slow the spread, as well. South Korea, for example, has been able to greatly control the virus by testing. They even have gone so far as to issue coronavirus bracelets so they can track infections. Now, that is just barbaric. I hope we never see that in the United States. However, there's really no reason that we can't do robust testing, as well—except for the fact that we were at the mercy of other countries selling us the kits.

We receive the lion's share of our drugs and medical supplies from about ten different nations. It's pitiful that all of the stuff is manufactured elsewhere, and the downside of that is now becoming obvious. The president should invoke the War Powers Act so we never have to depend on these countries again. We need tests immediately, because testing would need to be rolled out to the entire American population in order for it to be successful.

Ultimately, though, the whole calamity boils down to this: *This crisis does not end until there is a vaccine.* Until then, people can say whatever they want; people can take whatever path they want, or try whatever solution they want. It's all pointless, though. if there were something that worked, we wouldn't be discussing this. I can't be more blatant than that. Staying home or wearing a proper mask and keeping hands clean and washed is the only proven method of anything right now, until we get a vaccine.

In the meantime, what other actions should the government take to protect our citizens? First of all, President Trump was 100 percent right to pull funding from the World Health Organization (WHO). Why don't the complaining liberal elite just pick up the slack with private donations, if they think it's so important? Otherwise, China, Russia, Saudi Arabia, and others can foot the bill for whatever this rogue organization does anyway. We don't have daily briefings from the World Health Organization (The rogue WHO). In my opinion, all they do is take good money and make it bad money.

Regardless of what your belief is surrounding gatherings, pro sports, Olympics, political conventions, schools, and universities, there must be national uniformity for any belief to have merit. The only social experiments thus far are the NYC nursing home debacle proving elderly people die, and the pandemonium in the streets alluding that crowds of undocumented shoppers and other complicit individuals don't have a surge in death. The death rate to date in the US based on ANY date is just under 1 percent for all comers.

The timing can't be worse with the presidential election looming. I do believe the silent majority will give Trump a second term, merely to keep their taxes down, and anyone voting Democrat must know Biden suffers from dementia. Mail-in voting is instant corruption: if it looks and smells like shit, it's shit!

Taxes should be postponed. Just don't collect taxes for two years. Just say the IRS has closed for 2020 and 2021, and that's the end of it. Done, done done. This would be cheaper than the stimulus package, because it would not allow the Democrats to add every item on their wish list!

No property taxes, no income taxes, for two years. Just sign that into law. Why should people have to fill out application after application for a chance at money they'll have to eventually pay back? We're all in a crisis, and no matter how much we make, we're all living up to or beyond our means because we're stupid and greedy. We can't be taxed during a time like this. (If you're in the billionaire class, say starting with a net worth of five-hundred million and up, then maybe you do pay taxes.)

This would go so far. It really doesn't cost a lot to live, to drive around, and eat. It costs very little. The biggest expenses for most people are car and rent. With no taxes, and deferred debt payments, they could pay their rent. Small business owners could pay their employees.

Of course, the real solution is to eliminate our enemies. We need to shut all borders until we vet the good and sort out the bad . . . Let's not lose sight of the bigger picture and understand that this must be done immediately. (More on that in the next chapter.)

Ultimately, though, we need to find out why the CIA knew about all of this in January and did nothing. It's infuriating. Yes, China lied and withheld information, but it was obvious that something dangerous was happening. We should have been *expecting* China to lie to us. Instead of fighting back, we were totally asleep at the wheel.

What China did was to unleash a Trojan horse upon the world. They might not have intended for it to go this far, but they've managed to hit our nation in the kneecaps. Anybody who thinks that we aren't at war needs to wake up.

If I were the president right now, I'd be asking my smartest and most trusted advisors: What can we do to mitigate future risk of such a problem? How can we prevent or be better prepared for a future situation of biologic warfare? What strategy can be worked out perhaps with our closest allies for a global initiative against evil Axis governments that will always plague the West? As mentioned earlier, the Chinese fleet sailed past Japan on the way to Taiwan. This may be a dry run!

We need to stop China aggression, and I have a four-part plan to do it. One, we need to take back all jobs that can be done in the USA. Two, stop allowing foreign nationals to be educated here without extreme vetting. Three, stop selling debt to China and/or any adversary. Three, don't allow these communists to buy real property in this country without the most extreme vetting. It's time to look out for #1. When the forty million or so Communist Party leaders and families and friends with all their money come to the US and purchase real estate, they are driving up the cost of real estate for the rest of Americans. There's really nothing that's out of their price range. Not only does this keep Americans from participating in the housing market, but also it keeps American banks out of the lending business, because these people pay cash. Ultimately, that takes away American finance jobs. (This same principle applies to the Russian oligarchy and Saudi monarchs. They should be prohibited, too.) In the meantime, we should repossess the property they already own. They do it to us.

Fourth, and most important, we need to stop selling China US debt. The US debt to China is just over one trillion dollars. Lindsey Graham has suggested that we simply stop paying our debts as a way of punishing the Chinese. That is a bad idea. We cannot stop paying debt! Ten years ago, US debt was downgraded from AAA to AA+ because our GDP-to-debt ratio reached 75 percent. If we stopped paying our debts to China, our country's rating for debt would likely go to junk-bond status, meaning we could not borrow any more money, period. If we could not borrow any more money, the country would look no different from Detroit when they filed for bankruptcy. It would be an embarrassment and a disaster, surely one to incite no small degree of schadenfreude in the Chinese.

It is not that simple, Lindsey. We can't just stop paying back what we owe. We borrow money by creating bonds. We sell the bonds, and we pay the bond interest with taxes collected. We are already on the course to having escalated taxes beyond belief in the next few years because of this virus. There is no way around that. Anyone who thinks otherwise is simply in denial, clueless, or maybe venting.

Let me explain: If we assume just for the sake of round numbers that we have twenty trillion dollars in debt at the moment, and we just printed five trillion dollars more, we just made a 25 percent increase in our debt. By doing this, our debt payment goes from one dollar of every ten, to one dollar and twenty-five cents for every ten. The math is obvious.

So, there is a limit and a breaking point. Money cannot be printed indefinitely. We must honor our debts. The day we stop honoring our debts is the day we can no longer borrow money, which is the same as saying we can no longer sell bonds, and there would be no money for the country to function with. Instead of punishing the Chinese, this would be a course of action that would make them very happy, in the end.

China is our biggest problem. They are opportunists. Russians woke up and realized we can outspend them. After the fall of the Soviet Union, it became time for China to up their game. Boy, did they do that. We are facing a huge threat from them, and we need to take care of it. When it comes to China, if you're not part of the solution, you're part of the problem.

We are at war, and it's not a fair fight. There's never a fair fight. Anyone who thinks that anybody other than the United States of America follows anything from the Geneva Convention is really stupid. If you want to win a war and it means anything to you, how are you supposed to fight fair when nobody else does? It's time to start playing dirty.

CHAPTER 13
THE SOLUTION

To me, the world we live in began after World War II. People were in a hurry to make things better after the war, and everybody had a sense of urgency. Today, there is no sense of urgency, and nobody wants to make things better. They don't bother looking at what's broken to begin with. I do. This chapter may be hard for some people to read, but it's the truth—and accepting the truth is the only way to fix our broken healthcare system.

In the 1950s, being a doctor was a safe profession. People who didn't have family businesses encouraged their children to go into medicine because they were jobs that were stable and paid well. They wanted them to grow up somewhat affluent, but none of those people dreamed big enough, no one dreamed of billionaire culture. Comfort and safety for yourself and for your family were all that people needed—maybe with a nice car on top, too.

Back then, there were very elite, smart people still going to the US medical schools. Of course, there were pros and cons about that time. There was little diversity. There was a sense of entitlement. On the flip side, though, there was still an emphasis on learning and teaching, on building our professional class.

Old school values don't exist anymore. People have become too consumed with their lifestyle. Today, nobody takes any pride or care in what they do. They need to get home to their TV shows and TV dinners. The final straw, or perhaps where it started, has to do with the influx of foreign nationals. (I am not anti-immigration in medicine.) This is a huge problem.

If we want to save our society—which includes our medical system—there is a clear, black-and-white solution: Do not allow any more foreign nationals into our training programs, until we tighten the vetting process for all US-gained education. I'm talking about anyone who was not born and raised in this country. If you're Chinese and you were born and raised here? Come to Duke, John Hopkins, Columbia, Ursinus. If you're Indian American, and you want to go to Georgetown Law, Princeton, Brown, Northwestern, Stanford, and even Stony Brook? God love ya. (Shout out to Rik Mehta—a real constitutional conservative—currently running for US Senate from New Jersey with my full support!) But, if you're one of the fifty million who came overlooking for a better life than you've got at home? Well, I'm sorry, you *have* a country. Instead of escaping your country, you should be working to change your country. (I just love the people living here as permanent resident green card holders or even citizens who refer to other countries as their countries.)

Immigrants always like to claim that if they stay in their countries, they'll end up dead. They say that it's unfair to send them back to where they came from. Again, I'm sorry, but I'll say it again: Nothing in life is fair except the fare you give a bus driver. It's not our job to solve the problems of every other nation.

Sure, America is the melting pot, but people don't stop to realize that we've already done the melting. We made ourselves the most beautiful mix! You can go to Little Italy and get your fresh Italian pastries, and get your pierogis from the Polish Americans, and all of that is enough. The pot is full, and we need to take it off the burner before the pot overflows. Immigration, once a vital part of our country, has become a liability instead of a benefit at this point in time.

This should be so obvious, especially now as we deal with this pandemic. I am sorry if you're getting murdered in your homeland; you need to deal with your own government. Is it sad? Yes. Is it tragic? Yes. Is it horrifying? Yes. Do I feel the most empathy in the world for these people? Yes, I do. If I could help them, would I? Yes, I would, but I can't.

It's not going to help anyone if we let all their citizens in and turn a blind eye to what's happening over the border. Doing that means the degradation will continue forever, unabated. If we need to go over to discipline their countries to help their citizens, then fine, let's talk about doing that. Let's deal with the root issue. However, we cannot have an open-border policy that will only add to the welfare lines. This will not accomplish anything other than weaken *our* country and can lead to chaos and complicit activity. Current published estimates are 10 million illegal aliens (the real number is 30 million), and if allowed to stay, and they bring their families, the number jumps to 100 million. One hundred million people fighting for jobs with our citizens.

To the foreign nationals, I'm sorry. As I noted earlier, you cannot apply to school in the United States until we establish strict and thorough vetting protocols. We're not accepting you. It doesn't matter how much you bribe us. We don't need your money. We're the richest country in the world, and we learned that selling out to China for money is not worth the ultimate sacrifice—our liberty and freedom.

The foreign nationals who are already here should be vetted, like a global entry application and interview, too. If you're a foreign national of any country, 99 percent of the time you're a good person. But there is that 1 percent that is coming to our country to take our secrets back to God knows where, and we need to stop them. It would be one thing if they were coming here to be plumbers or fruit pickers, or something else that could help us. Instead, they're coming to steal our most delicate and privileged information, our secrets. It's just wrong. (And yes, we have homegrown problem people, too!—the government needs to spend MUCH more on mental illness-novel (new) therapies!)

Foreign nationals who have been living here ten or twenty years, however, should not be thrown out. They should stay in our country and keep on doing what they've been doing for their whole lives. I don't want illegal aliens getting money from the government and free healthcare. Why should they? That doesn't make sense. Whoever they work for should have to pay for their healthcare.

Ultimately, every real American citizen deserves to be able to make enough to feed their family. Having so many illegal aliens is preventing that from happening. However this heterogeneous society evolved, it needs to roll back up into its cocoon and it needs to come out different.

I'm not saying that any foreigners are inferior. In some cases, it is quite the opposite. Asians, in particular, are better trained than Americans. Chinese kids who have Chinese mothers are doing calculus when American kids are learning how to count. That's one place where we could take a cue from our enemies. So many American parents say that children need time to play and explore, but that's bullshit. You have an impressionable mind that can suck up tons of knowledge? That's the time to impart the knowledge (we need more polyglots).

Everyone needs to know how to add. Kids shouldn't even be allowed to see a calculator until they graduate college. Just recently, I was sitting there at the cash register, and I handed the girl a ten-dollar bill. I said, "The change is seven dollars and thirty cents." Instead, she had to put it all into the register to calculate it and the whole thing. I'm going, "Just give me seven dollars and thirty cents!" I get mad over these things, because it's like, these are the people who are supposed to pick up where my generation left off?

In addition to having basic math skills, every American child should be raised to speak two languages, at least. We should start teaching kids a second language from birth. I do NOT mean Spanish. Ultimately, that's not the most useful. We have nothing to fear from Mexico or Spain, for God's sake. Chinese would be ideal, because China is the real enemy. There are a billion and a half people speaking Chinese, so you would think it would be obvious that we should know it too, but Americans are just too lazy to take it seriously.

In the meantime, we don't need Chinese people who are born and raised in China, and want to live in China, to be educated in the United States. China needs to grow their own educational system and educate their own people with their own technology and their own science. We are not a country that should be disseminating our knowledge widely, because we are hated around the world, and we are a target. Don't you get it? There is not enough vetting in the world to prevent espionage in a situation like that.

Our enemies get it. Think about it: there's nobody born and raised in the United States taking microbiology courses in Russia or China. No Americans are studying nuclear physics in Iran. None. Still, somehow, it's no big deal when foreigners come here, learn everything we know from our best and brightest, and go back to building missiles they'll aim at us, or viruses that we can't cure.

When it comes to the healthcare system specifically, we have ourselves to blame for diluting the quality of applicants in medical schools. A void has been created by intelligent Americans going to work on Wall Street. Instead of medical school, these kids from top twenty universities are jumping straight into finance. With the changed standards, many patients complain that doctors speak broken English. The next time you have nothing to do— and coronavirus is not ravaging the nation—take a walk around a hospital with a blindfold on. See if you can decipher what is being said around you.

It's not just the fact that foreign nationals are taking American jobs that is the problem. These people do not share our culture and values. They do not know how to have an engaging, caring conversation with a patient. How is someone who was born and raised in Bangladesh and barely speaks English supposed to connect with and treat an elderly American who's terrified and in pain? They might miss important clues and cues because they don't understand the cultural subtext of certain statements. An individual should be not only versed in our language but our culture before they are let loose to treat patients within the American system. Foreigners entering the US for the long haul should speak our language and adopt our customs. If they choose not to, I would question why did they leave their homeland.

To truly change medicine, however, *everything* in our country has to change. That much should be clear by now.

When it comes to politics, for example, we must eradicate the concept of the "career politician." Nobody should be entitled to a second term, because the minute you get in, you're already distracted by your run for the next term. Nobody should have more than one term, and there should be no exception to that rule—not even the president.

A presidential term in today's world should be six years, and that's it. The second change to happen at the White House is the federal government has to pay the president a fair salary. You have to pay the president, say, billions of dollars a year, and they must pay taxes on that. It's taken for granted that you don't pay rent at the White House. It's taken for granted that you don't pay for your food. You don't pay for your clothes, or your flights—*if* your travel is for true official business. If you're on leisure time, you should have to pay for your own security and your own travel. President Trump could really drain the swamp once and for all if he would commit to this kind of plan. God knows that he of all people could afford it. If it doesn't start at the top, how the hell can it filter down?

The next change that the government should enact would be to allow medical professionals to use the government's prenegotiated rates with vendors. Everyone knows that innovative drugs and treatments are increasingly expensive. Oftentimes, insurers refuse to reimburse doctors at a fair rate.

One disturbing example comes up while treating scleroderma. In the 1970s, a scleroderma patient with a hypertensive renal crisis would die, unless they had bilateral nephrectomy. Today, ACE inhibitors, such as Captopril, are used to completely control this condition. Captopril comes in 50 and one 100 mg tablets. Fifty mg is the indicated maximal dose for hypertension, while 100 mg is the maximum dose for heart failure. However, a scleroderma renal crisis requires that the dose often be raised to 700 or 800 mg daily to work, thus exceeding the package insert dose maximum. Guess what. Even though the drug is generic and has been around for decades, insurance companies will not allow it to be covered at that dose without a lengthy phone call that has to go through multiple clerks and other paper passers. We have to fight to be reimbursed for the extra cost.

A problem we face as physicians is dealing with bureaucracy. The federal government allows appropriate testing and procedures. Sadly, if you are hardworking and turn out in the top 10 percent of billers within your specialty—making too much money or seeing too many patients—you could be (the top 10 percent of billers ARE) targeted for an audit. Hence, medicine is socialized and will criminalize you. At the same time, private insurers are denying most testing at an alarming rate merely to save money. They should understand that older drugs have multiple uses and package inserts are not fully accurate or up-to-date. I find it ludicrous that I run behind with my schedule trying to engage in peer-to-peer phone calls to appeal on behalf of my patients, when I have yet to speak with a peer on the phone. It is typically a nurse or midwife, not my PEER. This is a regular occurrence. If your appeal is successful with the insurer, they will find other ways to delay you longer. And it will delay proper patient care for weeks or months or longer. The solution is less government regulations and auditing, and less policing of appropriate doctoring from the private sector.

The problem is, we can't just hop the border to get cheaper prescriptions in Canada and Mexico, like our patients do. If any doctor were found to be doing that, he'd find himself or herself in jail. Meanwhile, the government has low, prenegotiated wholesale prices with drug and medical supply vendors, known as the "government rate." That rate should be accessible to all healthcare professionals. If it's good enough for the VA, why can't every hardworking man and woman benefit? Trust me, it's not going to hurt the drug companies. They sell to the government at half-price and still manage to make a tidy profit. Truly, the amount of money that these companies are hoarding is disgusting. The less they wine and dine doctors, the more the CEO takes home. More jobs weren't created for innovative scientists, sadly.

When I started my career thirty years ago, the drug companies wasted millions of dollars on dinners, cruises, gifts, trips, travel, ball games, elaborate meals, clothing, watches, jewelry, and so much more on buttering up doctors. (Was it really a waste? Are all doctors on the take? We weren't paid to do any wrongdoing, merely taught about new products.) If you spent any time with them, everything was included. Doctors used to line up to give lectures for the drug company, because they'd pay you anywhere from two thousand to five thousand dollars for a forty-five-minute talk. It was a good gig for doctors, until the federal government passed the Sunshine Act in 2010. Now, all of this has been taken away. I'm not complaining; I can pay for my own vacations. I *am* asking, however, where did all that money go? Where did the "butter up the doctor's budget" get redirected? Curious why other lines of business can be treated nicely by vendors in their designated professions, including politicians.

Speaking of those good old days, I'll never forget a fishing trip that I went on with a drug rep who is a good friend. (Over the years, as a large account I made the careers of many pharma reps by my shear volume. My reps become VPs and higher. We grew together with hard work.) He decided to take me out deep sea fishing, and five minutes out of the harbor, I'm puking my guts out. The captain refused to turn the ship around, so the guys are all up on the deck fishing and drinking beers while I'm practically dying below deck. Finally, I had enough. I snuck upstairs and dumped all the bait overboard. Fishing trip over. The captain finally turned the boat around, and as soon as I hit dry land, I was ready for lunch.

Those days are gone, however, and the money that used to go to deep sea fishing hasn't disappeared. It must be somewhere, and it should be utilized. All drug companies with revenues in the billions of dollars should be required to direct profits to research and development for conditions that have no sufficient treatment. Instead of beefing up their 401Ks, the drug scions should be trying to find cures for conditions like Alzheimer's or cancer, just to name a few.

Moreover, they should be banned from developing drugs in the same class of drugs that they already sell. For example, they should not be allowed to create more beta-blockers, NSAIDs, or TNFα inhibitors *ever*, unless we find a cure for every type of cancer and every unusual condition that exists on this planet. (Basically, never.) There should not be patent extenders. If a drug expires after twenty years, it's done. You can't relabel it and sell it under a different name.

We could solve all of the world's health issues, but we're not prioritizing correctly and putting people over profits. Why do we need Motrin, Advil, Excedrin, *and* Aleve? They shouldn't even be produced. They're wasting money. Drug companies will spend millions or billions just to create Motrin under a new name, when they could have made a billion dollars by creating a novel drug for a disease that doesn't have a cure at all. (Not to mention, they'd be saving millions of lives; but let's not kid ourselves that that's what they're in business for.)

These companies should be mandated to manufacture entirely in the United States, even if it costs more. Basic rule of thumb: You get what you pay for. Now this is coming back to bite us. Greedy CEOs using what I would equate to slave labor in China or Mexico to save a few bucks have created a system that is not sustainable. In particular, it is urgent that all American companies remove their jobs from China in as rapid a manner as possible. This will ultimately destroy China. We should take back our jobs from other countries, too, while we're at it. It may cost these companies more, but in the long run we will all be better off.

We need to just accept that we are not the best at everything and go from there. The fastest man in the world is not from the United States. He is from Jamaica. We have to apply this rationale to making parts. Maybe there is someone in China who can do it better, faster, and cheaper. Sorry, but he needs to stay in China and work for his country. We need to cultivate from within and promote Americans from within. That may not be optimal, but it's something we must learn to deal with because it is better for us in the long run. Small businesses deal with this all the time, and small businesses do everything better than the US government. This has nothing to do with any administration. It's the inherent lack of foresight demonstrated by lifers in the government and imitated by greedy CEOs. Short-term losses caused by bringing jobs home should be thought of as long-term investments in the American economy.

When we are able to revive the American economy, one underserved area that these companies could focus on would be genetic engineering. We need to implement genetic engineering in this country on a much larger scale. We've done everything we can to try to outsmart Darwinism, and look where it's gotten us. Now, we should think about letting nature do its work: rather than targeting individual diseases that are genetic, I would prefer to see effort and money spent to solve the entire problem through gene modification for all genetic disorders. Perhaps in the process the lazy gene can be identified and eliminated.

Anyone who knows me would tell you that I am really compassionate, and I help everybody. Even though I'm so busy, I treat loads of people for free. I can't buy somebody ten thousand dollars' worth of drugs every month, but I can certainly do free office visits, free X-rays if somebody has no money. So, I do.

You can believe me or not, but sometimes Archie Bunker is right. If people had listened to some of the things I've said over the years and implemented them, we'd be in a much better place. First of all, can you imagine what our country would look like if we'd stopped welcoming in our enemies in droves?

It just makes sense: You don't destroy a country that hates you just to rebuild it. It's not normal. You don't send your jobs to another country; you just don't do that. The more we fill our residencies or training programs with midlevel providers and foreign-born graduates, the more we are diluting what was once the world's most elite healthcare system.

Meanwhile, the system as I have described it is only getting worse. If it keeps getting worse, there will come a point where doctors will simply start dropping off, or they will stop going into medicine. Nobody went to medical school looking for a nine-to five-job that pays as much as a desk job. For the past one hundred years, the smartest people went into medicine so they could get a measure of respect from society and they could earn an above-average paycheck. No doctor was ever expected to become a billionaire, but all doctors expected to make a million dollars over the course of their careers.

Unfortunately, today's graduates are looking for that million-dollar check before they start working. They are planning their calendar before they plan their patient hours. How do we change this mindset?

Well, for one, doctors need to be paid fairly in a free-market society and be allowed to make as much money as they can. The busiest doctors are the ones who are going to provide the best care, keep patients out of the hospital, and make sure that their health is in check. Those patients will cost the system the least amount of money. In return, those doctors will see more patients and perform whatever procedure is unique to their specialty. Ultimately, they will make a lot of money, which will make them happy.

This will allow the smartest, most ambitious people to resume the pursuit of medicine. Hopefully, doctors will regain the respect that they used to engender.

What role will other medical professionals have in this system? While midlevel providers and medical assistants have very different roles, some medical assistants are smarter than the doctors they work under. (Thank you to Denise and Dana, who have both been with me for more than twenty years!) These people are literally invaluable and can be paid as much money as they choose. Everyone should be fortunate enough to have an innovative, self-motivated genius as their medical assistant. I, for one, have been blessed in that way and cherish my medical assistants above most other doctors I know.

Nurse practitioners or physician's assistants assume a role very similar to that of the doctor, but various doctors will utilize assistants in different ways. While some doctors have the assistants do paperwork, others have them assist in surgery. Some of us train them as well as we can, essentially making them into above-average doctors. We let them operate on their own and perform patient visits that are of the same quality as those of a trained physician. (Of course, in such cases I will stick my head in the room at the very least, to make sure the patient knows that I am still involved in their care.)

Again, it is a blessing to find this type of individual, and doctors should empower them to succeed. It only helps the entire system overall. Of the dozen or so that I've trained, all stayed in the field of rheumatology because my methods of teaching are very exciting. (You can see for yourself on my popular YouTube channel and social media feeds.) It is fabulous to see the excitement in people's eyes and words when they learn what is really happening in medicine.

In fact, one of the greatest pleasures that I have encountered in my professional career has been training nurses and others in the field of rheumatology. One of my former nurse practitioners—who never even heard of rheumatology until meeting me—is now regarded as one of the top rheumatologists in Virginia. She has trained the physicians that she joined, as she was well ahead of their knowledge base because of what she learned and absorbed directly from me.

Tim Lieske is another young medical professional whom I have mentored. This is his story, in his own words:

> Dr. Soloway's office is unique in that he has an X-ray department. Because he has an X-ray department, he is part of the radiology program at the college that's down the street. When I was a student, I did a rotation through his office, and when I graduated, they hired me.
>
> I was really young, twenty-four, and I was kind of shy, so I was intimidated by the doctor. He's my boss. When I talked to him, it was pretty much all business. I've been there sixteen years now, so a lot has changed.
>
> He's been a great role model and father figure for me. He'll have all these people in the waiting room, and he's constantly calm and just so driven. Watching him over the years taught me, I just gotta fly straight.
>
> At one point, I even got into some trouble, and Dr. Soloway gave me a second chance to turn my life around. A lot of people wouldn't have done that, and I'll never forget that he did. I have a great life today, and a lot of that is due to him.

Then, there's Julia Tillman, who joined my office as a teenager and was able to pursue her nursing degree on the job:

> In his office complex, Dr. Soloway used to rent out space to another doctor. I worked for them part-time. Then, there was a Quest lab inside of his office complex, which my mom ran for, many, many

years. Between going back and forth to school, my afterschool program, my co-op, and work, I would run by him and say, "Hey, Dr.
Soloway!" I always thought he was great.

Then I got laid off of my job. I happened to be at the lab with my
mom one day, and he said, "Hey, do you want a job?" I said, "Yeah,
it couldn't hurt!" That was fourteen years ago. I started working
for him when I was nineteen, and I'm thirty-three now.

I always thought Doc was great. The office is always busy, and it
can get stressful, but he's always been more than great—always
very polite, mannerly, and funny.

You know, I've always looked up to him as a father figure. He's
wonderful. He'll listen to you and heal any problem you have. If
you're ever overwhelmed, you can just go and talk to him. He's
always very calming with what he has to say. Like, "It'll be all right,
just do what you can."

Throughout the years, he's been more than wonderful. I went to
nursing school and it was a lot, and he worked with me. He let me
adjust my schedule, work the weekend, catch up on my work. He
would sit there and help me practice my clinical, whether it be
taking manual blood pressure or just anything. He was just
awesome.

For me, our office has always felt like a family. I'm never afraid to
talk to Dr. Soloway about anything. If I have an issue or a problem,
I'm never afraid to text him, email him, or even just say, "Hey, I have
a suggestion." He's always, always open ears, super accessible. He
even just randomly checks in with you to make sure everything's
good, like, "If you need anything, just let me know." He's great.

Ninety-nine percent of our patients absolutely love him, too.
The only complaint I've ever heard is the wait time. I tell them,
"Look, you can wait six months to see him or you can wait the four
hours to get fit in the schedule that day. You're going to wait for
one day versus six months."

There are so many patients who say their quality of life is so much better after seeing him. They're more active. They're able to go back to work, and it's amazing that this is what he does.

He always puts his patient first. There's never anything about money or anything like that. He's just focused on taking care of them. For example, every day we order gourmet sandwiches for lunch for the patients. There's a whole bunch of different kinds of hot chocolates and coffees. They have access to snacks, a whole refrigerator full of drinks. It's a very comfortable setting, not like a hospital or a nursing home. It's a great place to be and he's just awesome.

Of course, my absolute favorite medical mentee has been my own daughter, Alyx Soloway. This is her story:

My dad has been talking to me about writing a book for my whole life. It's so funny that it's finally happening!

My earliest memories of him were by his side in the office, when he used to bring me along to meet with patients. I would stand in the corner while he would give the injections, and I was terrified of needles. He would always tell me something like, "It doesn't hurt. Just talk to him about something you like. Talk to them about ice cream!" While he would inject someone's knee, I would sit there and talk to people about shakes, sundaes, their favorite ice cream flavor. When he was done injecting, they were all really happy. I'd probably have said it was because I talked to them about ice cream.

Now, we work together at his practice while I'm finishing my medical school. [She has graduated and is an internal medicine resident.] It's a blessing and a curse because he is the exact same person off-duty and on. People love him or hate him, and sometimes it gets him in trouble. He adapts to his audience, but his humor is really that of an eight-year-old boy, and that is going all day long. He has a wonderful staff who really support one another, and they joke around all day. Even though you have angry patients who are waiting forever, everyone is happy and smiling. It's a very positive environment, and a lot of the people who work there have been there over twenty years, almost since I was born.

Getting to be able to work alongside him has changed our relationship forever. As a kid, you don't appreciate the hardworking parent because they're not who you see every day. As a kid, I definitely was angry that I didn't see him as much as I thought I should. He'd be working late, or working on a Saturday, and I was like, "Well that's great, dad, but I'm here and I'm waiting for you. Who's more important than me, you know, as your daughter?" I didn't understand, but I get it now. It took me a while to get here, but I just get it.

Because I've been working at his office, I understand that the reason he's late all the time is because when someone really does need his help, he drops everything to help them. If it takes two minutes or two hours, he will sit there and figure it out. A normal doctor might tell you, "Look, I have all these people waiting. It's been twenty minutes and we're out of time. Make another appointment." My dad really is committed to sitting there all day if it takes that and figuring it out. As a patient, of course, you really appreciate that. As a kid who's waiting at home for him, I'd just get mad.

There are some patients who get mad too, but if you had a problem, wouldn't you rather have him sit with you and figure it out, rather than write you off? There's always someone, at least one person a day, who needs at least an hour from him.

The other factor in his work is that instead of referring you to everyone under the moon, he'll figure it out himself and do this whole workup for you. He really takes a different approach. It's the right way, the forgotten approach. He treats the whole patient, even if their problem doesn't necessarily fall under rheumatology.

The most important lesson I've learned from him is that you don't treat lab tests. You treat people. It doesn't matter what the labs say, and it doesn't matter if they confirm or deny your suspicions, because your clinical judgment is way more important.

The second-most-important lesson would be to give the patients the time that they need. If it's a simple case and you can run in and out of there knowing that you did everything necessary, then you do that. But, if it's a complex patient that people have been ignoring for forty years and this person is still in pain, you need to take the time and figure it out.

I've seen people come in completely, debilitatingly crippled and he diagnoses them without even looking, because he is so used to it. Quite frankly, at this point I could probably diagnose them without looking, too, if I asked the right questions. Then, in a month or two they're so much better. They sit and wait three hours just to tell him how much better they feel and how much they love him, and how appreciative they are. It's almost shocking that no other doctor was ever able to do that.

He just really, really cares. When I started shadowing him at the office, I was very upset because he was running three hours behind. I said, "Dad, it's really distressing that you run this way. It bothers me."

He started tearing up, and I'm like, "Oh, God. Like, what did I do?"

He goes, "Alyx, I never want to disappoint you. You try so hard, and I never want you to be disappointed by what I'm doing." He was so hurt to think that I wasn't proud of him, or that I was disappointed.

People like Alyx, Tim, and Julia give me hope for our system's future.

What does that future look like? Without further ado, here's how we fix the healthcare system. First, please understand that any vision I could possibly have would take at least fifteen years to institute. The pendulum always swings—or so it seems—but it took us thirty years to get to the problem state that we're in now. It will take at least fifteen years to get out of it.

We currently have somewhere between ten and fifteen health insurance companies in the United States. They all have various fee schedules, and doctors negotiate various rates with these insurance providers. On the other hand, as discussed earlier, Medicare is not cost-efficient at all. It pays doctors the least, audits the most, and creates ongoing hassles for doctors. Ninety percent of Americans have health insurance, while ten percent do not. Of these 90 percent, two-thirds have private insurance through their work or pay for it themselves. Americans should have the choice for what's best for them.

If an employee has been vested long enough to get 401K or pension money, they should also be vested to receive health insurance through their employer. Small businesses should get a tax credit to be able to pay for employee health insurance. People would be insured, and companies would see an increase in employee gratitude, loyalty, and work ethics. This is part one of fixing the healthcare crisis.

Until Americans have filled the lion's share of medical jobs, foreign nationals should enter a lottery based on merit to fill remaining spots. We should always feed our own first, and focus on quality should be of utmost importance.

Doctors should be able to avail themselves of government rates when it comes to supplies and drugs. Drug companies should invest in treatments for underserved conditions instead of replicating existing products.

Politicians should be limited to how long they can serve, and how much pension they can get. No one should ever mention the words "Medicare for All" ever again.

Finally, of course, everyone—without exception—should get themselves a kick-ass rheumatologist.

CHAPTER 14
RHEUMATOLOGY FOR DUMMIES

The waiting list to come see me can be intimidating, and beyond that, not everybody wants to come visit Vineland, New Jersey. For that reason, I've built a solid following on YouTube, where I post informational videos and full lectures. I have 200,000 views, and more than 5,000 followers on Facebook, and 2,500 subscribers to YouTube/stephensolowamd.com.

Whenever someone posts a question in the comments, I do my best to answer it. I've had questions from other medical professions from Afghanistan to Zambia, and one hundred countries. These are some of the most commonly asked questions, from the very basic to the very advanced:

Arthritis

What is arthritis?

Anything that ends in "-itis" means inflammation. Tendonitis is inflammation of a tendon, for example, while chondritis is an inflammation of cartilage, and arthritis is an inflammation of a joint. Then the question becomes, what's the joint? A joint will be one of two types. There is the standard diarthrodial joint, which is the elbow, for example. Then, you have the standard ball and socket joint, like the shoulder or hip. Basically, a joint is when two bones come together. They are separated by cartilage and connected by ligaments so they can move. The space that makes the joint is surrounded by a fluid called the synovium. When the synovium is inflamed, you have synovitis. These are all very important terms when it comes to arthritic conditions, known as a class to the lay person as simply arthritis.

How does the synovial fluid come into play, and how does that help you under-stand what's going on inside a joint?

Normal synovial fluid looks like water. It's clear, but it's more viscous than water. Its main constituent is hyaluronic acid, which is a thick gelatinous material that serves as the water in the fish tank, if you will. The synovial fluid has all the nutrients to take care of lubrication and nutrition, because the cartilage between the bones of the joint doesn't have a blood supply or nerve supply. The synovium does have a blood supply, so we rely on the synovium to provide a living environment for the joint.

In disease states, we get problems with the synovium, and the nature of the fluid can change. You can stick a needle into a joint and take out synovial fluid to help with diagnosing. The fluid you extract could be blood. It could be cloudy. It could be yellow and cloudy or yellow and clear. It could be white. It could look like toothpaste. The analysis—both grossly and micro-scopically (light, dark, and polarized microscopy)—will tell you if there is a fracture. If you see lipid droplets in the fluid, it can be indicative of fracture in the case of a history of trauma. If there is no history of trauma, it could be pancreatic disease. If you see cholesterol plates, they are often indicative of chronic bursa effusions. You can tell if there's an infection in the joint by looking at the organism under a gram stain or having it grow at a lab. You can see if an artificial joint is loose by the presence of cement particles. More generally, you can understand if a condition is inflammatory, versus simply wear and tear. In those cases, a determination depends on how many white blood cells there are in the fluid.

If you get recurrent blood, not only could it be an injury, but you can diagnose diseases as rare as scurvy, because Vitamin C deficiency causes hemarthrosis, or bleeding in the joint. There's so much to be learned from looking at synovial fluid.

Sadly, there is no orthopedic surgeon that I've ever met who has any idea what to do with synovial fluid, except to order someone else to examine it. They only do one test, which we don't even consider to be standard: a Lyme PCR. They believe you can diagnose Lyme disease from the synovial fluid, but you can't. You diagnose that by a blood test and by the exclusion of everything else.

How do you diagnose which kind of arthritis someone might have? Just from the synovial fluid or a combination of factors?
Everything is in the history. Historically, what's important is when did it start? How many joints are involved? Are the joints symmetric? Are they asymmetric? Are they large joints, or are they small joints?

Large joints refer to wrists, elbows, shoulders, hips, knees, ankles. Small joints refer to any of the knuckles or toes. They also refer to the acromioclavicular or the sternoclavicular joints, which are two of the three shoulder joints. Although people aren't aware of it, the sacroiliac joints in your pelvis also count, and you can drain fluid from them. Typically, we don't talk about the facet joints, which are the spinal joints, because we generally put needles in them for pain relief rather than for draining stuff.

What if they don't have a history? If somebody comes in for the first time, can I diagnose them based on their presentation? For example, somebody comes in with one joint that's red hot, tender, and swollen; sudden onset with no injury; no trauma. That person probably has a crystal arthritis, meaning gout, pseudogout, or another crystal. If they're a dialysis patient, that might include hydroxyapatite or oxalosis.

On the other hand, say somebody comes in with anywhere from two weeks to six months of pain in four or more different joints across the body, such as right ankle, left knee, right hip, and two fingers on the opposite hand. That would be asymmetric oligoarthritis, and the differential diagnosis for oligoarthritis would tend to include any of these common conditions: ankylosing spondylitis, psoriatic arthritis, the arthritis of Crohn's disease, the arthritis of ulcerative colitis, the arthritis of hepatitis C, the arthritis of sarcoidosis, the arthritis of celiac disease, or the arthritis of Whipple's disease. Sometimes you might even see that pattern in reactive arthritis.

If somebody comes in with a small joint *symmetric* arthritis—which means, on the same side—the diagnosis would depend on which joints are affected. For example, if you make a fist, the knuckles that are closest to your elbow, not the ones closest to your nails, are called the MCPs: metacarpal phalanges. The bones that are on the top of your hand, those are the metacarpals, and then you have the proximal phalangeal, then a joint, then a distal phalangeal, then a joint, then the nail. If somebody comes in with symmetric swelling or arthritis or synovitis of those MCPs, now you're talking about a differential diagnosis altogether. That would include rheumatoid arthritis, lupus, or hepatitis C.

Now, some of those can overlap, because they have different modes of presentation, such as chronic sarcoid arthritis, psoriatic arthritis, chronic gout. Gout could go in the oligoarticular arthritis category, as well.

To play devil's advocate, if somebody has enlargement of those MCP joints but does *not* have synovitis, meaning they have wear and tear of those joints, then you have to think about hemochromatosis or calcium pyrophosphate deposition disease.

Now, if we move down to the two knuckles, the one adjacent to the nail and then the one in the middle, the one next to the nail is the DIP or distal interphalangeal joint. The one in the middle is the PIP, or the proximal interphalangeal joint. In people over forty experiencing pain there, my conclusion would probably just be osteoarthritis, which is by far and away the most common arthritis. It's often genetic or from wear and tear. It's often very painful, but unlike rheumatoid arthritis, the history is that there's pain with use. It's not pain with rest.

A correct diagnosis involves looking at location and size of joint. When does the pain occur? In the case of gout, or crystals, it's acute, explosive onset without trauma.

Osteoarthritis is use-related pain. That means, I'm sitting in the chair and when I get up, my knees are stiff for five minutes. If my knees are stiff for an hour and a half when I get up in the morning, that's inflammation. If the inflammation is only in one knee, it can be anything from an infection to every single solitary thing that we named—and stuff that I didn't name.

I'll throw in one curveball. What's unique about hypertrophic pulmonary osteoarthropathy? It looks inflamed, but it's bland, and it's associated with lung cancer.

Then there's acute sarcoid, also known as Lofgren's disease. The patient comes in with swelling, synovitis, warmth, tenderness of both knees. It could be going on for a week, a month, or six months. The ankles have periarthritis, meaning tendons, ligaments, and everything else that's inflamed, not just the joint. The joint may be involved, but when it's everything else, that's acute sarcoid. In addition, that usually comes with a rash, fever, and shortness of breath.

How can people know when stiffness or pain crosses the line into something a doctor needs to look at? What would you tell people?

I would tell them, the more you pay me, the better answers I'll give you (lol). In all seriousness, the moment to see me is when it starts to interrupt their quality life, or two weeks of symptoms. Another important flag is a change in the pattern of your pain. If you've been living with your pain for ten years, and all of a sudden, Monday, things are so bad or things are so different that you just don't understand it, you should see me. If you develop new pain in any joint for no reason that doesn't go away on its own within three to five days or a week, you should see me. That would go for any joint. If it's red, hot, and swollen, you need to come immediately, because we want to make sure it's not infected.

What if there is someone in their thirties with no presenting issues at all. Are there any signs that they should look out for as potential early warnings of future arthritic problems?

The most common cause of monoarthritis in a woman in her thirties is gonorrhea. It shows up as monoarthritis (one joint), and it's usually the same presentation that could occur with Lyme arthritis. It's usually a knee, with gonorrhea. Gonococcal arthritis creates a couple of interesting challenges. One, it's extremely difficult to diagnose because even if the joint fluid is pus, the organism only grows 50 percent of the time with chocolate agar.

If it's not pus, it will grow the organism less than 50 percent of the time. You have to base your conclusion on clinical suspicion, or a vaginal exam. DGI, or disseminated gonococcal infection, is the unifying diagnosis when the vaginal infection of gonorrhea spreads out of the pelvis and can involve the joints or skin. It gives what's called hemorrhagic bullae, which is the typical rash, and it gives arthritis typically in the knee. You have to treat it with antibiotics, and you also have to treat for concurrent chlamydia.

Back to your original question. The indicators that you could look out for would be joint stiffness that's out of the ordinary for you. Remember the old phrase: If you stand in shit long enough, you can't smell it. Don't be one of these people who suffers through years of pain and just thinks it's normal. It's not normal. It's especially not normal just because you're getting older. Don't use age as an excuse to explain pain.

People might be afraid of getting a diagnosis, but the cause of your pain or someone else's pain doesn't have to be a malignant or malicious outcome. If you have pain, go and check it out with your arthritis specialist; not your orthopedic surgeon, your rheumatologist. That said, I may be the only rheumatologist that'll give you the right answer.

People who are younger, especially fit people, tend to think that pain is caused by degeneration or an injury. How should they know to come to you versus going to see a physical therapist or sports doctor?
Let me give you a great example. Larry Bird's career came to an end because he couldn't run or jump anymore. The team doctor, who was an orthopedic surgeon, after treating him for several years, finally got him to a rheumatologist, where they said, "Oh, you have psoriatic arthritis." They treated it, and he was fine, but nobody recognized that the tendonitis he had wasn't because of basketball. It was actually inflamed tendons. The spondyloarthropathies, of which psoriatic arthritis is one, are often associated with tendonitis of the heel, Achilles, ribs, sternum, or back. Psoriatic arthritis ended his career, but if it had been diagnosed immediately and treated immediately, his career would have lasted longer.

If somebody has pain with prolonged morning stiffness or inability to perform the activities of daily living, that person needs to come immediately. You can't just attribute it to playing sports.

A similar phenomenon is that people probably in their forties and fifties start to have back pain and think it's an old sports injury, or an inevitable part of aging. What do you say to them in terms of which kind of treatment they should pursue?

When people get to that age, that's when symptomatic osteoarthritis starts to occur. Osteoarthritis is caused by wear and tear, or genetics, or both. Old injuries do come back to haunt you. People typically have back pain, or they have knee pain. They have trouble with grip strength. Thinning of the cartilage occurs. The bones get closer together, the motion gets more minimal, the tendons and muscles around those areas get stiff. As you get older (over forty), you need to stretch more because if tendons get stiff you lose motion, and with lack of motion you lose strength.

The typical first steps to easing symptoms—which is usually what people have tried *before* they see me—includes heating pads and Tylenol at a thousand milligrams, three to four times daily, which is the maximum dose depending on your age. That can be mixed with NSAIDs, which are things like ibuprofen products.

Other treatments could include physical therapy, stretching, chiropractor, back support, acupuncture, yoga, Pilates, or swimming.

When they get to me, it's a highly precise injection to the joint or tendon sheath that gets rid of the joint pain. In the case of the knee, you also can inject it with reprocessed, normal joint fluid, also known as hyaluronic acid. Likely works in all joints; insurance typically doesn't pay for hips, shoulders, etc.

When should people with age-related arthritis think about coming to see you? Should they come early or until Tylenol's not enough and it's unbearable?

If you wake up in the morning with pain, you're going to pop an Aleve and stretch and hope it goes away. If it doesn't go away after that, you're going to alter your exercise routine. If that doesn't work, you're going to see your chiropractor or GP, and they'll give you a prescription for Celebrex. That won't do anything.

If you have pain for more than a week or two, you need to come see me. If you were taught how to strengthen your joints properly, you could probably cope with it better in the long run. I would never say you could "stop" the arthritis, because that's not currently possible. However, if you learn proper exercise techniques, you can greatly minimize your suffering.

I recommend isometric exercises, as opposed to isotonic exercise. Isometric exercises can strengthen the muscles around your joints without actually moving the joint. Planks are an isometric exercise, for example. Strengthening your muscles in that way can help deflect some of the weight-bearing from the joint to the muscle. That's never proven to halt the progression of the arthritis in a literal sense. People are happy when they actually follow that protocol. The same goes for a knee brace. Knee braces can be amazing depending on who, what, where, why, when. For example, if somebody's symptom is that their knee occasionally gives out, you get them a stabilizer brace and it can't give out.

Seeing a doctor immediately upon the occurrence of a problem is beneficial, whereas putting it off and waiting until later puts the doctor at a disadvantage. The person who's got the pain may just assume it's part of aging, when in fact they might have one of the inflammatory conditions and would never know otherwise.

What about an area such as the hip? When people start to have pain there, is it generally osteoarthritis or something else?
When someone comes in and says, "My hip hurts," my response is, "Can you please put your finger where the pain is?" If their finger's in the front, then that's the hip joint. If it's on the side, that's the trochanter bursa. If it's in the back, it's either coming from the lumbar spine, the gluteal muscle, the piriformis muscle, or the posterior of the hip proper.

That's just a rough outline. If it's literally in the very front, it can be ilio-pectineal bursitis, which is the bursa that sits on the hip. If it's on the outside of the leg, 99 percent of the time it's going to be trochanteric bursitis. However, it also can be iliotibial band syndrome. When it comes to "My hip hurts," in most cases that's not going to land an arthritis diagnosis.

That will lead to a true, true, and unrelated scenario. What's a "true, true, unrelated scenario"? A patient comes in, says, "Doctor, I have knee pain. I got hit by a car and it ran over my neck. So, the accident caused my knee pain." Yes, you got hit by a car. Yes, you have a bad knee. Sorry, they are not related, and you can't get disability based on this information.

In another example, say that before they got to me, they had an X-ray of the spine. Because they're over forty, that X-ray showed arthritic changes. Unfortunately, however, they don't know that it's *not* osteoarthritis that's causing those symptoms in their hip. It's true that they have arthritis in their back; it's true they have pain in their hip; the two are not related.

It's very important to understand which abnormalities are actually asso-ciated with symptoms, as opposed to being normal age-related changes. You could have a back riddled with arthritis and scoliosis, but if it's not hurting, it's irrelevant.

On the other end of the spectrum, what is the youngest patient you've treated?
Of the several dozen kids whom I've seen under the age of ten, most have been between the ages of three and seven. Arthritis in children is known as juvenile arthritis, although the exact wording often changes.

There are different patterns to look out for. The most common is a blonde blue-eyed girl who's around five years old and has a positive ANA (antinu-clear antibody). Typically, they don't complain of pain. Instead, the mom notices they can't play or ride the bike. They crawl instead of walk. So, the mom notices it but they don't complain. (This is very important, because a child complaining of pain often has leukemia.) They're usually very shy at the office, but you can see clearly that they have inflammation or swelling of a joint. It's usually a knee, maybe an ankle, maybe a wrist, or an elbow. The one good thing about the condition is generally they will outgrow it by age sixteen. However, they absolutely are treated like adults from onset until it burns out.

They must get an eye exam every three months because it is associated with uveitis, which can lead to blindness. You start them on ibuprofen. If the ibuprofen doesn't work within a week, you give a little prednisone and you put them on a TNFα inhibitor, which is a biologic. You give them a self-injectable, and the mom injects at home. Methotrexate is often used—typically a biologic gets used.

There is another form that occurs more in boys starting around age seven or eight. They tend to get one of two things. One, they get an onset of rheumatoid arthritis young; or two, they start off with pauciarticular arthritis, which affects two to five joints. (In adults, it's called oligoarthritis.)

Polyarthritis is six or more joints. It looks just like rheumatoid arthritis in adults, and it's treated in the same way. If it comes along with fever and swollen lymph nodes, then they call it Still's disease. Again, it's treated with interleukin inhibitors as opposed to TNFα, but they're still under the category of biologics. They're often very sick, but they're also very treatable, and they sometimes burn out, but not always.

Juvenile arthritis often occurs with a small jaw (micrognathia) with fusion of the cervical spine. This must be differentiated from psoriatic arthritis, because psoriatic also can fuse the cervical spine, and so can ankylosing spondylitis. However, the fusion in ankylosing spondylitis or psoriatic arthritis has to be differentiated in the teens or twenties, not at ten years old or twelve or fifteen.

How much of arthritis is genetic, as opposed to lifestyle-based?
Let's focus on two categories to answer the question, because in each case the answer is wildly different: inflammatory arthritis and noninflammatory arthritis. Noninflammatory is the forty-year-old who's got arthritis in the knee, the thumb, or lower back. Lay people refer to noninflammatory arthritis as "the good kind." It is the most common form of arthritis and often has

a genetic predisposition. There's no question about it: "My parents used to have hands that look just like that!" I hear it all the time. It's so generic, and it happens to be genetic, too.

Of course, there are environmental factors involved. If you're a librarian, you're probably going to have less wear on your joints than if you're a mason or a pro athlete. A laborer will wear out faster than a librarian.

The "bad kind" of arthritis—at least in the eyes of the public—is the inflammatory or rheumatoid kind. Rheumatoid is not the most common inflammatory kind of arthritis. Gout is. Gout affects 5 percent of the population, while rheumatoid arthritis affects 2 percent of the population.

Spondyloarthropathies—such as ankylosing spondylitis, the arthritis of Crohn's disease, ulcerative colitis, and psoriatic arthritis—probably occur more frequently than rheumatoid arthritis, as well.

In terms of the "bad kind" of arthritis, we need to split it into two further subdivisions. Column A includes rheumatoid arthritis and lupus. Column B includes psoriatic arthritis and ankylosing spondylitis.

For Column A, there is a genetic predisposition. You have billions of particles of information in your body, inherited from your mom and dad. If you inherit a sequence that puts you at risk of getting one of those conditions, then as long as you come in contact with an environmental stimulus—which is currently unknown—it'll turn on a switch (I'm not talking about pheromones!) that will likely give you one of those types of arthritis. Large populations of rheumatoid arthritis patients happen to be positive for a genetic marker called HLA-DR4.

When it comes to Column B, psoriatic arthritis and ankylosing spondylitis, they are linked with a marker called HLA-B27. It is said that 100 percent of people with ankylosing spondylitis are HLA-B27 positive. I don't know for sure if that's 100 percent accurate, but it's certainly 99 percent if not 100 percent. With psoriasis or Crohn's, it's probably on the level of 50 percent, but it's still a tremendous percentage. (Although HLA-B27 negative, 70 percent of celiac patients have sacroiliac involvement.)

While this is not diagnostic, say somebody between twenty and sixty years old walks into the office, and they tell me, "My left knee and right heel have been swollen for like nine years." I'll talk to them, get their story, and find that part of their differential happens to include psoriatic arthritis.

I'll ask, "Does anyone in the family have psoriasis? Parents, siblings, only blood relatives."

They say, "Oh yeah. My mom and her mom and her mom and her mom, they all had psoriasis." Well, that person has psoriatic arthritis. You still have to do the blood test to make sure they don't have something else, but you can go to the bank with the fact that they have psoriatic arthritis until proven otherwise, with or without HLA-B27 positivity. Fifty percent of the time, though, it will be positive.

Autoimmune Diseases

Recent studies have claimed that autoimmune diseases are on the rise in our country. Is that true?

First, what is autoimmunity? Autoimmunity means that the body attacks itself. With more use of rheumatology comes more diagnosis of what we treat!

The bone marrow makes white blood cells, red blood cells, and platelets. Platelets and red blood cells are just happy being by themselves. White blood cells come in many types; the more common include neutrophils, lymphocytes, monocytes, and eosinophils.

Neutrophils—also known as polys—typically fight infections (through the process of phagocytosis), while eosinophils are typically seen in asthmatics or in people with allergies or parasitic diseases. Monocytes are seen with infections. Finally, lymphocytes.

Lymphocytes are the most confusing. They have to differentiate into B cells and T cells. B cells and T cells have a commensal relationship. If an intruder (antigen) enters the body, then the antigen presenting cell greets the intruder at the door. The antigen presenting cell processes the antigen. It becomes memorized to your database, so it can be fought off if it's seen again (memory T cell).

Depending on the antigen will determine how they differentiate, and they'll recruit other cells. In the case of autoimmunity, it's the lymphocytes.

Plasma cells (these are the cells that produce antibodies), are mature B cells, that when overproduced, lead to a category of diseases referred to monoclonal immunoglobulin deposition disease. One within my field is amyloidosis. Amyloid protein is associated with deposition in joints. Oddly enough, the shoulders are uniquely involved.

The lymphocytes that attack the nucleus of our own cells are known as antinuclear antibodies (ANA).

When you measure a patient's blood to test for the presence of ANA, if it's positive, the possibilities are almost endless. I'd want to find out: Is it an autoimmune disease, such as RA, lupus, Sjogren's, scleroderma, or myositis? Is this a nonrheumatic autoimmune disease, such as Hashimoto's, myasthenia gravis, pernicious anemia, or immune-mediated polyneuropathy?

Testing for ANA is the gold standard when it comes to testing for autoimmune diseases. The proper testing is the Hep-2 cell assay (an indirect immunofluorescence assay). Other techniques are not sensitive or specific.

Many labs do not titer (an amount) past 11280. The lab I use will "titer to end point."

The first positive is called 1:40. You take two drops of bleach and you put it in, it's still blood red. The second one is 1:80; three, 1:160; four, 1:320; five, 1:640; six 1:1280. If you don't get the point by now, I give up.

ANAs rise with age. One can speculate over time, you come in contact with more environmental stimuli, viruses, or other unknown antigens that stimulate autoimmunity. It may follow that if people live to older ages, of course more people are going to test positive.

I think the major cause in the rise of autoimmune cases is that the population is growing, and environmental issues such as pollutants, chemicals, and viruses are rising, too. The other factor is, now you have family doctors, GPs, and Urgent Cares order a superfluous ANA as part of their screening, when in the past, rheumatologists only ordered them when they had suspicions that a condition was present. (That is what we refer to as pretest probability.)

For example, if somebody is seventy and they have a positive ANA, a rheumatologist would generally say, "Well, who cares? It doesn't mean anything. What were their symptoms? Why did you order the test?" (Because the pretest probability was low.) Depending on the symptoms, one might change their viewpoint.

If somebody comes in saying, "All my joints hurt. I have a rash. I have a fever." In that case, you have to consider all possibilities. Your differential diagnosis would include, but is not limited to, lupus, Sjogren's, scleroderma, myositis, rheumatoid arthritis, and more. The antinuclear antibodies can be seen in all of them, and usually are. You can still have an autoimmune disease even if the ANAs don't show up on the test. As a doctor, however, your confidence in your diagnosis goes up as the ANA titer gets higher. If I see an ANA of five thousand, ten thousand, or forty thousand, this is indicative of a problem. From there, you just have to solve the problem.

With a number like that, I just know that the patient has *something*. From there, it's my job to correlate it with the other autoimmunity tests to see which pattern they fit. If the ANA and double-stranded DNA test are both positive, that's a lupus pattern. If ANA, SSA (Sjogren's Syndrome A, or anti Ro), SSB (Sjogren's Syndrome B, or anti La), and rheumatoid factor are positive, that's a Sjogren's pattern. If they have myositis-specific antibodies (antibodies seen in inflamed muscles), or synthetase antibodies, those people typically have inflammatory muscle diseases. If the person has ANCA (antineutrophil cytoplasmic antibody), that's vasculitis-associated. There are then different types of vasculitis depending on the different patterns of the ANCA, which is often seen with vasculitis. ANCA is to vasculitis what ANA is to lupus or rheumatoid arthritis.

You can have a classic rheumatoid arthritis patient who's got a positive rheumatoid factor and CCP (cyclic citrullinated peptide) antibody. CCP is more specific than rheumatoid factor when it comes to diagnosing RA. For example, if the CCP is greater than two hundred and fifty, then they have RA and you don't even have to think. However, if it's between forty and eighty, they definitely have something, and it's probably not RA unless their rheumatoid factors are really, really high, you've excluded other causes of a positive rheumatoid factor, and the patient has a small joint symmetric polyarthritis. Rheumatoid factors are seen in many, many, many conditions, though. The most common of those conditions would be lupus, Sjogren's, scleroderma, and hepatitis C.

Gout

What are the most common signs of acute gout?
The sudden onset of atraumatic redness, tenderness, warmth, and swelling. Together, those four adjectives comprise the definition of inflammation.

Say someone's feet just started swelling and burning. Could that be acute gout?
The sudden onset of atraumatic explosive pain could be the whole foot, one joint, two joints, three joints, the skin, the tendons, or any combination of that. There are no rules, and most joints and organs are not spared, when it comes to gout. The heart valves aren't spared. The vertebrae aren't spared. Gout can affect any joint, or connective tissue.

Most cases of acute gout—from 80 to 90 percent—only involve *one* joint, however. If *both* feet are swollen, that's edema, which would be caused by heart failure, a slow thyroid, liver failure, or too much protein in the urine.

Sudden atraumatic swelling is a sign of gout. How long does the swelling associated with gout normally last?
The natural history is seven days. Without treatment it should go away in approximately seven days. It comes back later 90 percent of the time; once you've had an attack, you really need to start planning to keep chronic gout state under control.

For people with gout, that means keeping their uric acid low, typically with the uric acid-lowering therapy Allopurinol. The typical cutoff is 6 mg/dL, but I don't think six is really acceptable because there's a lot of fluctuation in testing. It's the same as jumping on the scale five times, and it says one hundred nine, one hundred eleven, and one hundred seven. I like to give it leeway just in case and aim for the lower the better.

Let me make this clear, however: gout is not diagnosed by any blood test, including the serum uric acid. It can be suggestive of it in the correct clinical scenario. In the correct clinical scenario, we call this clinical, but not crystal-proven gout. (Clinical gout means the story sounds good, and then you don't have a better explanation.) Crystal-proven means you saw the crystals, so you've proved it. Ultrasound, which is gaining popularity and is becoming widely used (mostly for the purpose of raising one's income) is considered more and more to be acceptable to diagnose gout. I disagree with this, because there are many examples where it cannot prove anything, i.e., there can be more than one condition, and the presence of classic gout on imaging doesn't equate to the current pain being from gout! It can't exclude an infection in the face of gout. It cannot exclude mixed crystals in the face of gout, and more.

Another example is if somebody has a hot, tender, swollen joint. If you drain the fluid and you identify crystals inside the white blood cell, this is a guaranteed diagnosis that gout is causing the inflammation. Using ultrasound, you might be able to prove they have gout, but you cannot prove that the event actually occurring at that moment is from gout.

How does crystal-proven diagnosis work? If you have something that's inflamed, whether it's skin, tendon, or joint, stick a needle in the inflamed area. You will come out with something on the tip of the needle, and you make a wet prep and examine it under your microscope. The positive identification of a gout diagnosis is made by the identification of monosodium urate crystals. If you happen to get lucky and see a monosodium urate crystal within a white blood cell, this confirms that the attack at hand is related to that crystal.

When a patient has a swollen knee, finding crystals shows you that they're a gout patient. It doesn't tell you that the inflammation is due to gout. To determine that the attack at hand is from gout, you must see phagocytosis with a martini sign (the crystal is seen in the WBC, or white blood cell). Did you know that you can have severe gout in an artificial joint? If you're not aware of this, refer to my article in the *Journal of Clinical Rheumatology*. If that's not enough, did you know you can have CPPD in an artificial joint, too? If you're not aware of that, you can find my article in the same *Journal of Clinical Rheumatology*.

After diagnosis, how do you treat gout?
There are two types of treatments: the treatments for the acute gout, and then the treatment for chronic maintenance. For acute gout, the treatment is merely to get rid of the inflammation. For chronic care, the goal is to lower the uric acid as much as you can, with an absolute highest max of six mg/dL (milligrams per deciliter).

There are two ways to lower uric acid: one is to dissolve it, and one is to help push it out of the body. The mainstay of treatment is Allopurinol, which dissolves it. If Allopurinol is not effective for any number of reasons, we now have Krystexxa (pegloticase), which is a uric acid-specific enzyme. Humans do not have uricase, which breaks down uric acid. By using Krystexxa, we are giving the body an enzyme it does not have, and that breaks down the uric acid very effectively. Many doctors do not prescribe Krystexxa, because it is very expensive and given intravenously. I would equate it to Remicade for RA.

If you have a patient who's had chronic, severe, refractory gout, you keep them at zero for a year or two. In that time, you'll dissolve away most of their gout crystals, and they'll go from looking like a corrugated box to normal skin. I've seen it happen. The results are profound.

A lot of doctors could struggle with patient compliance when you require intravenous treatment twice a month. My solution has been simple: if you miss a treatment, we don't take you back. That's gotten me 100 percent compliance.

The healthcare system should be thanking me for that, by the way. I've saved the insurance companies so much money by controlling patients, because they are almost never referred to the hospital.

Gout was known as "the king's disease" and is often thought to be caused by eating rich foods. Is that true, or is any of it genetic?

Gout is a metabolic disease. More than 95 percent of gout patients are under-excretors of urate, likely due to a renal tubular defect. The few people who are overproducers of uric acid either have an enzyme defect, a malignancy, or even something like psoriasis.

Back in the old days when it was known as a rich man's disease, people were just eating themselves into oblivion. Gout is often associated with metabolic syndrome, which is a combination of hypertension, diabetes, hyperlipidemia, and gout. It is common.

Which kind of lifestyle changes do you recommend to gout patients?

The number one lifestyle change I recommend for gout patients is coming to my office, if they don't already know me.

There are some foods that are actually protective when it comes to gout. For example, red wine and dairy foods are protective against gout, while beer and organ foods, sardines, and anchovies are provocative.

Other than that, I tell the patients that if you want to lose weight, you need a healthy lifestyle and a healthy diet. My typical advice is just that: a healthy lifestyle does include an hour of exercise a day built into it. Putting that aside, flip back in the book to the section where I describe a healthy diet.

If someone doesn't take care of their gout for years, will it get worse and worse, like RA?

Chronic gout is actually very hard to distinguish from RA, because the appearance on the outside looks identical. That's when you have to get blood tests and try to stick a needle into a joint to identify gout.

Do you see gout more frequently in men or women?

Gout is far more common in men than women. Men's uric acid rises at puberty, while women's uric acid rises at menopause. Historically, women prior to menopause don't get gout, and historically men prior to puberty don't get gout. I've seen exceptions to both rules. It's common that men get a first attack in the toe or the ankle, while it's common that elderly women who take water pills and baby aspirin get it in their knuckles.

Low-dose aspirin elevates uric acid, which is why these women get gout. High-dose aspirin, formerly used to treat rheumatoid arthritis decades ago, lowers uric acid so much that patients treated for RA years ago never had gout, and it's only recently that we realized that the two coexist, since we don't use high-dose aspirin in the treatment of RA anymore. Out of my cohort of six hundred patients, twelve had tophaceous gout, with RA.

What is the newest advancement and/or best treatment currently for gout?
The newest treatment is Krystexxa (pegloticase), which causes a rapid and dramatic drop in uric acid. This allows for the more rapid dilution of the gout salts that are deposited throughout the body. It works so well that it cleans out gouty deposits that have been left in kidneys, heart valves, and any other parts of the body. Most noticeable is when tophus are dissolved from nodules under the skin and you can actually watch them go away.

As long as it stays at zero, you are dissolving this stuff faster than the speed of light. Then, it passes through the body and gets peed out. That's awesome. In fact, many people don't know this, but their renal insufficiency or kidney trouble is often due to the tubules being clogged up with gout. In my experience, I've seen several patients' kidney function improve 20 to 30 percent on Krystexxa (pegloticase).

You would think every rheumatologist would be jumping on this, but I'm still an outlier. Krystexxa came out five years ago, and as of three years ago I was the only one using it in New Jersey. I got a lot of heat for being ahead of the curve—the only rheumatologists routinely using the drug are at Duke University, where they did most of the clinical trials.

Lupus

What are the initial signs of lupus?
Initial signs can be anything, but wide-ranging, the most common being

rash or arthritis. In addition, you may see constitutional symptoms, such as fever, night sweats, weight loss, lethargy, malaise. However, I've seen patients present solely with proximal muscle weakness, pleurisy, pericardial effusions, and nephrotic syndrome, which is one of the kidney issues. I've even seen people present with Raynaud's.

Who is the typical lupus patient? I really don't know if there is a typical lupus patient.
Often a young black woman with renal involvement is the nightmare scenario. The most common is inflammatory arthritis or photosensitive rash and abnormal blood tests. The female-to-male ratio is nine to one. Blacks have a higher prevalence than whites, and young black women under twenty-four years old statistically have a worse prognosis than old white men. In spite of the ratios, I have a large number of patients who are white, black, Chinese, Hispanic, and in every decade of life from twelve years old through the nineties.

Most commonly, I see lupus with kidney involvement, or other life-threatening lupus in all comers. For example, I recall one lupus patient who presented with Raynaud's and ended up losing several fingers. She did have phospholipid antibodies, as well.

What's the youngest that you've ever seen?
I saw a young white boy of eleven years old with lupus nephritis. It's reported that under five years old this does not occur. You never say never, but these are some general rules that we follow.

Are there other conditions that people might mistake for lupus, or vice versa?
Viruses or cancers are commonly mistaken for lupus. Infections such as tuberculosis can mimic lupus. However, the real trick comes to decipher other connective tissue diseases from lupus. These include myositis, sarcoidosis, Still's disease, Sjogren's syndrome, relapsing polychondritis, ANCA vasculitis, and IgG-4 related diseases.

Sometimes making a diagnosis of lupus can be difficult, because not all the features need to occur at the same time, and they may occur over months, years, or a lifetime, and blood tests are not always reliable.

Lupus patients have arthritis that for all the world looks like rheumatoid arthritis, and in either case they may be associated with fevers and constitutionality. In either case, they may have pleurisy or hemolytic anemia, leukopenia, or lymphopenia, which is low white blood count. They might have low platelet count, which is thrombocytopenia, or hemolytic anemia, which is when there are antibodies against the red blood cells. That causes people to be anemic.

Regarding some of the mimics, sarcoidosis is a great mimic. Sarcoid is differentiated by the presence of noncaseating granulomas in the biopsy.

Sjogren's syndrome, Crohn's disease, and lymphomas are mimics, as well.

Raynaud's can be a primary or secondary condition. Primary is simply a young woman who has a reversible spasm of the blood vessels, the arteries, the arterioles, the smallest blood vessels. It's characterized by anywhere from five to sixty minutes of the so-called triple phase color response where the fingers or other body parts go from white to blue to red. This is often precipitated by stress or cold temperature. If there's no associated disease, that would make this primary Raynaud's. If Raynaud's occurs in the setting of another disease, it would be referred to as secondary.

The same thing is said for keratoconjunctivitis SICCA (in English, dry eyes and dry mouth). Dryness of the eyes is diagnosed by that which is severe enough to cause corneal damage. Dry mouth is typically quantified by a salivary gland biopsy, in which the lymphocyte score is greater than one lymphocyte focus per four millimeter squared.

Another mimicker is adult-onset Still's disease, which is characterized predominantly by sore throat, lymphadenopathy (swollen, nontender lymph nodes), hepatosplenomegaly (enlargement of the liver and spleen), and fevers that spike and go back to normal every day (quotidian fever). Lupus can look like this also.

Finally, there's what's referred to in rheumatology as pulmonary renal syndrome, which is when a patient presents with inflamed lungs and kidneys simultaneously. The short list for things that do this include lupus, cryoglobulinemia, and ANCA vasculitis.

With so much overlap, how can you make a definitive diagnosis of lupus?
A definitive diagnosis of lupus is made by characteristic clinical findings and supportive lab data or biopsy. Supportive lab data include positive ANA and positive double-stranded DNA (ds-DNA), and Smith antibodies (Sm, not to be confused with smooth-muscle antibodies, which is abbreviated SM).

Typical biopsy findings would include direct immunofluorescence staining for complement or immunoglobulins.

Lupus remains a *clinical diagnosis* unless supported by biopsy findings and positive serologies (see blood tests above). Clinical diagnosis of lupus is usually defined by the presence of the correct antibodies or biopsy. Research criteria have been established and typically change every ten to fifteen years. These criteria are not in any way suggestive of how one should treat patients with suspected lupus, whether or not they fulfill all the criteria.

The lupus criteria are solely for research purposes—not for diagnostic purposes. It really depends on how you want to explain it to the patient.

Say the patient comes in and they have a constellation of symptoms or events over a lifetime. For example: "Last year I had pleurisy and I was in the hospital for a week and nobody knows why. There was the time my joints were hurting for like a year and they were swollen and stiff for an hour every single morning. Plus, somebody said I had Raynaud's. Somebody else said it could be rheumatoid arthritis, but it went away. So I didn't really deal with it," and blah, blah, blah. Finally, something else happened, so they got evaluated. Somebody checked their blood and threw in the ANA test.

If the ANA is positive, that finally gets them a referral to a rheumatologist. From that point, the rheumatologist goes ahead and orders the double-stranded DNA test, and the Smith antibody. If you have a positive ANA with a significant titer and you have a positive double-stranded DNA or positive Smith antibody, then that person has lupus. Period. End of story. (However, if the blood was ordered randomly and the person has no symptoms, then there's no disease to treat that's visible—meaning to say, there is no treatment that will prevent the onset of lupus.) It's not 100 percent, but there's nothing that's more specific. Unless you can come up with a better explanation, that's it.

Various medications cause positive ANA. They typically don't cause positive double-stranded DNA. They do cause positive single-stranded DNA and positive histone antibodies.

While the value of ANA is not diagnostic of any condition, the higher the titer, the more likely it is to have an association with a disease process.

Now for the impossible situation—even for the best. Imagine going to the supermarket and shopping for a dozen eggs. You open the container and only find a dozen yolks. This is the equivalent of finding a positive DNA with no positive ANA. When this lab anomaly shows up, we generally are as confused as you would be, and we often just rely on our best judgment and experience to figure it out.

Markers of increased disease activity in lupus include elevations in double-stranded DNA, or decrease in complement levels. The value of ANA is not recognized to correlate with disease activity. Although it is positive and need not be positive a second time. Sometimes, it is repeated inadvertently.

The DNA is high when the disease is active, and lower when it's not—sometimes. This is a barometer, which is not very accurate but is used nonetheless. You need to take it with a grain of salt, like so many things.

Feckless physicians tend to rely on blood tests more than clinical evaluation. There's no justification for continually checking tests. (It is important to monitor chemistry, CBC, and urinalysis to look for medication toxicity.)

If you have a positive ANA with double-stranded DNA, or an ANA and Smith, along with an associated disease, you likely have lupus.

One quick crib note: If there's a patient with pleuropericarditis, we often say it's cancer, TB, or lupus. Why can't it be RA? It can't be RA because RA usually presents with joint pain and pleural effusion, or joint pain and a pericardial effusion—not with both. Lupus *can* do both, while the other similar conditions usually don't.

Another example is dry eyes and dry mouth. Is it lupus or Sjogren's? The ANA and the SSA are both positive, nothing else. If the ANA is 1:640, and there's a positive SSA, that doesn't fulfill the criteria for anything. One doctor might tell the patient they have lupus (in spite of what I just said). Another might say it's Sjogren's (again, in spite of what I just said). Which is it? At the very least, this patient has autoimmunity, and it would appear that they have an overlap of lupus and Sjogren's, but since they don't have the criteria for either or you still can't differentiate one disease from the other, they are said to have an unspecified tissue disease.

It's a matter of looking further. With dry mouth, do a salivary gland biopsy. If the biopsy shows a lymphocyte score of one focus of lymphocytes per four millimeters squared, this is a positive test for Sjogren's. In a Sjogren's patient, you're not going to see any immunofluorescence.

Finally, when you're comparing glomerulonephritis (kidney inflammation) in lupus versus vasculitis, lupus nephritis gives typical immunofluorescent staining of IgG and complement, where ANCA vasculitis reveals pauci immune deposits. In either condition, patients can have pulmonary hemorrhage, chronic sinus infection, nosebleeds, and pulmonary renal syndrome. On the surface, either one could look like Sjogren's or lupus.

Testing such as a CAT scan of the paranasal sinuses can be helpful.

If you're not confused yet, then you need to keep reading over and over again, because lupus, Sjogren's, and vasculitis can all look the same, and subtleties within lab testing or biopsy solve the question most of the time.

Clearly, there is a lot of overlap where these diseases are concerned. It might be hard for people to be labeled with the correct diagnosis if they're not working with a specialist in the field, a rheumatologist.

Anecdotally, it seems like there are more cases of lupus in recent years. Has testing improved, or what's going on?

Testing is very standardized. Most labs correctly use the Hep-2 cell assay, and rheumatologists are very comprehensive in their testing. More people are aware that for the proper diagnosis of these diseases, they must see a rheumatologist, and this may lead to more diagnosed cases when they were previously undiagnosed cases but were ill nonetheless. Don't forget, the insurance company forces a diagnosis. If almost close or similar, it may just be a label for the insurance company to pigeonhole things.

This is no different from a million people allegedly having coronavirus when a small percentage of the population has been tested. Once everyone has been tested, we'll know the real number.

Rheumatologists ask themselves, what is the pretest probability of a patient having a positive test? If the pretest probability is very low, you probably shouldn't order the test. If the test is ordered and is a low value, then the patient probably does not have an illness. If your pretest probability is high, then a positive result is consistent with your thoughts and more indicative of the problem at hand.

As people age, ANA positivity occurs more frequently. The specific reason for this is not altogether known. However, if octogenarians all have positive ANAs, don't go looking for a lupus outbreak. If an octogenarian is in the hospital with pneumonia, under normal circumstances ANA does not need to be ordered.

To play devil's advocate, a medical student might ask, "Can you prove this isn't lupus pneumonitis?"

"No, I can't prove it, but the patient doesn't have lupus, so why would you think that?"

"Well, if you can't prove it, can't you just check the ANA?"

If the ANA comes back positive with low value, that would probably be a false positive, so now you've created confusion for someone with no experience in that field.

One bit of trivial information: It's been suggested that rheumatologists tend to have positive ANAs at a higher rate than the average population.

Perhaps this is due to the fact that we are constantly exposed to people with a multitude of diseases with unknown causes or stimuli.

Two of my mentors died of Lou Gehrig's disease, and I always found that peculiar. Even though Lou Gehrig's disease or ALS is a neurologic disorder, I think there must be an immune-mediated process. Could that be related? There's no proof of that connection; just speculation.

What causes lupus? Is it all genetic, or are there lifestyle factors involved?
The cause of lupus is the body's attack on itself, otherwise stated as anti-double-stranded DNA. Hormonal issues play a role, as noted by the higher prevalence of females to males, the exacerbation with estrogen and clotting in lupus patients, the deficiency of DHEA-s (also known as DHEA-sulfate). Environmental factors include exacerbations from the sun.

What are the best treatments right now?
Current treatments for lupus, whether indicated or off label, include but are not limited to the following: NSAIDs, Plaquenil, Cellcept, cyclophosphamide (cytoxan), methotrexate, Imuran, Benlysta, IVIg, DHEA-sulfate prednisone.

For some of the drugs that weren't mentioned, here are some other reasons to use lupus drugs:

Alopecia—topical JAK inhibitor
Lupus profundus—dapsone
Alveolar hemorrhage—Cytoxan dosed one or two milligrams per kilogram daily
Prevention of heterotopic ossification after hip replacement—Indomethacin

I just named close to fifteen drugs, yet only three drugs, plus Benlysta, are approved: aspirin, Plaquenil, and prednisone. (That was the indication back in 1950.) It's so hypocritical that drugs are allowed or disallowed based on their price, when it comes to off-label usage.

It's universally standard that all patients are on hydroxychloroquine, also known as Plaquenil. Hydroxychloroquine has proof of lessening lupus flares, clotting, and renal flares and lowering cholesterol in lupus patients. You can have a patient who is stable on nothing else but Plaquenil for the rest of her or his life.

When someone has a flare, however, what do you do? The general answer is to give them steroids. Beyond that, however, it depends on the organ that is flaring.

If somebody has lupus of the kidney (lupus nephritis), you're going to give them pulse steroids 1 gram 3 times daily. You may or may not use cyclophosphamide, and you will probably use CellCept, which is also known as mycophenolate mofetil or MMF. If you use those medications, it works. CellCept does not have an FDA indication for lupus, but anybody with lupus of the kidney is on CellCept—just like Plaquenil—and they do just fine. CellCept does not have an FDA indication for lupus; however, it is the standard of care!

If someone has a flare of muscle disease, pleurisy, pericardial disease, or arthritis, you're going to start with oral steroids in a lower dose. If it's arthritis, you're going to probably add methotrexate. You're going to be left with CellCept long term, along with maybe some steroids, or not.

You definitely use Plaquenil for lupus skin disease, and you need to push skin protectants as much as possible: Don't go to the beach, wear sunscreens, wear protective clothing. They're possibly going to need a mild topical steroid on certain parts of their skin, depending on how bad the rash is.

Psoriasis

Can you diagnose psoriasis just from clinical presentation, without any further testing?

Yes. Psoriasis has moved from a dermatological disease to a rheumatological disease, since the treatment is generally guided by rheumatologists. Furthermore, 15 percent of skin psoriasis patients get the arthritis of psoriasis, also known as psoriatic arthritis. There are five different varieties of psoriatic arthritis—none of them good. (Actually, there are six, but it's anecdotal only. It's a PMR presentation of psoriatic arthritis, which I've seen in 1 percent of one thousand people over thirty years.)

However, all of them are easily treatable with biologics. (Speaking of which, Phil Mickelson, call me if you want to get your psoriatic arthritis treated by the best!)

The most natural treatment for psoriasis is sunlight, while newer therapies called biologics, namely TNFα and interleukin inhibitors, are excellent in more severe disease. TNFα inhibitors or interleukin inhibitors are excellent particularly in combination with methotrexate, when treating moderately severe psoriasis or psoriatic arthritis.

While psoriasis loves the sun, lupus hates the sun. Psoriatic patients hate the winter, and they love the summer. Lupus patients are just the opposite.

When someone has psoriasis, do they tend to go to a dermatologist first?
People still go to a dermatologist first more often. However, with each passing day, more people are more aware that this is becoming the domain of a rheumatologist, who is the one more aggressive with the treatment.

Twenty-five years ago, if an individual had psoriasis, the likelihood of their coming to your office? The answer would be never. Now, in my opinion, 15 percent of people who have psoriasis come directly to the rheumatologist. (It's because all their friends told them it's treated better by a rheumatologist.)

What is the best treatment for psoriasis?
The biologic drugs (TNFα inhibitors or interleukin inhibitors) are best in the treatment of psoriatic arthritis or psoriasis, with or without methotrexate added. In my opinion, all biologic drugs work better in combination with methotrexate than without.

Even the worst patients can be remitted 100 percent. These patients go from looking like they're covered in wet cement mix to looking completely normal in three to six months. In fact, there are patients who get their first infusion, and when they stand up, there's scaling on the chair.

We have people literally with total body coverage, almost 100 percent. The person who has a small scale behind their ear would never seek physician advice. I'm only seeing the most severe cases, so my standard of care is to use medications indicated for severe disease immediately. In the patient population I see, there's no such thing as a "wait-and-see" approach. The results are mind-blowing.

Kim Kardashian, a very vocal psoriasis patient, seems unable to control her psoriasis. Do you have any thoughts on the matter?
While I've never met and don't know anything about Kim Kardashian, I go back to basics and say that assuming there's adequate patient compliance, if somebody with a common disease and good treatment is not doing well, one needs to look again at the diagnosis and the treatment, because one is wrong. I'm the best. If she would come see me and would follow my directions, I would be able to control her psoriasis. (Ms. Kardashian, please feel free to call for an appointment.)

Patients take it upon themselves to read the package insert, which is loaded with fear. They need to take the advice of an experienced clinician who sees thousands of patients to understand which side effects are relatively common, and which are unheard of, but need to be listed.

What other conditions besides psoriatic arthritis can include psoriasis?
Although psoriasis is a skin disease, it can cause arthritis, tendonitis, nail changes, dactylitis, and enthesitis (the enthesis is what connects a tendon into the bone). Enthesopathy is a cardinal feature of this condition.

The five types of psoriatic arthritis are: mimic of rheumatoid arthritis, DIP and nail involvement, arthritis mutilans, sacroiliac disease and axial arthritis, and large joint oligoarthritis. (This could sometimes be considered the sixth type: In the twelve hundred patients whom I have diagnosed with polymyalgia rheumatica, or PMR, twelve patients or 1 percent in fact have psoriatic arthritis, and I propose that a patient can have psoriatic arthritis that presents as PMR. These data have never been published.)

Spondyloarthropathy

What is ankylosing spondylitis?

Ankylosing spondylitis is the Cadillac of spondyloarthropathies. It is an inflammatory disease of back pain that involves the sacroiliac joints and the spine. It involves peripheral joints, most commonly the hips and shoulders. It is not limited to the joints. It involves enthesis, tendons, and extra-articular manifestations that include cardiac involvement, pulmonary involvement, and involvement of the eye. A variety of other organ systems are involved as well. The disease affects men more than women. It is typically diagnosed before the age of forty. Its onset is always before the age of forty, and usually much younger than that. Women usually have a worse course and/or prognosis than men. There is a strong genetic predisposition to HLA-B27: 100 percent of patients with ankylosing spondylitis possess HLA-B27, while 10 percent of the caucasian population of the United States is HLA-B27 positive with no disease. There are geographic tendencies, as HLA-B27 is not observed with regularity in sub-Saharan Africa. In the most northern latitudes, HLA B27 occurs in 100 percent of particular Eskimo tribes.

Dactylitis, which involves swelling of a digit, typically a toe, refers to a digit that resembles the shape of a sausage, presents lots of visibility of the wrinkles in the skin, and has inflammation at all levels between the skin and the bone, including but not limited to tendons, muscles, and fascia. This is very characteristic when identified by the physician. The X-ray findings of ankylosing spondylitis are indistinguishable from the X-ray findings of Crohn's disease or ulcerative colitis.

What's the difference between psoriatic arthritis affecting the back (axial skeleton) and ankylosing spondylitis?

While both are fundamentally the same, the major differences include pattern and distribution of the sacroiliac joints and the spinal column. The sacroiliac joints in AS are bilateral and symmetric. The same goes for the spinal column: cervical, thoracic, and lumbar. Psoriatic arthritis typically involves unilateral sacroiliac disease with asymmetric disease of the spine. Ankylosing spondylitis tends to have more prevalence of other organ involvement. On the contrary, the X-ray findings of Crohn's colitis are indistinguishable from those of ankylosing spondylitis. That said, they all look about the same!

One of the diagnostic tests that can be abnormal in either condition is a technique known as the modified Schoeber's test. This reflects limitations in lumbar flexion.

What is the best course of treatment for spondyloarthropathies?
It's the same as treating psoriatic arthritis: biologics. There is nothing other than biologics that will help axial disease. I like to treat them with a TNFα inhibitor and methotrexate combined. I do believe that the combination of methotrexate and TNFα inhibitors works better than methotrexate or TNFα inhibitor alone.

If you have a person who's got early ankylosing spondylitis, and they present with ankle or elbow swelling—not the back—methotrexate alone will work for their symptoms. Steroids can be started, and it will simmer down the inflammation quickly.

If you give patients this treatment and they're not better in six months, you really, really better question the diagnosis, check the dose, and check that it's being given correctly. That is one of the reasons that I prefer infusible drugs over subcutaneous drugs, because you can force compliance 100 percent.

Everything in the vein works better. You get better distribution of the drug, better penetration. You don't have to worry about the possibility of not absorbing 100 percent of the drug. You don't have to worry about an old stomach or a stomach with gastritis or esophageal reflux causing any issue.

Letting people do subcutaneous injections at home can cause many issues. I had a patient who lost his hip and knee because he injected through his clothing. He told me his pants were clean when he injected, so he didn't understand what the problem was—definitely not the brightest thing to do. The infection was totally out of control, but he did not think that cellulitis of the whole leg was a real issue. He waited two or three months to tell anyone about this problem. It could have been avoided with IV.

Ever since I started using IV biologics, the side effects that I see are minor: maybe positive ANA or minor cases of drug-induced lupus. Drug-induced lupus won't kill you. You get a rash and feel like crap and then you realize it started three months after you got on Remicade. So, you stop the Remicade and you give them something else.

If you have them on methotrexate to start, though, it will block those antibodies and prevent the drug-induced lupus.

A lot of jealous doctors have accused me of administering IV medication just to make money. This is a horrible accusation, and my enormous patient population would tend to disagree with any of these haters.

Patients with axial involvement are recommended to be in a swimming program or a yoga program to help stretch out the spine.

Finally, the last question: Dr., do I have the good or the bad arthritis?
The good arthritis, osteoarthritis (a.k.a. OA), is typically a function of wear and tear or aging or possibly genetic and typically causes pain controlled by Tylenol or local joint injections. The bad arthritis, known as rheumatoid arthritis (a.k.a. RA), reflects inflammation with destruction of the joints and surrounding structures, which is known as the crippling arthritis. It happens that over the past twenty-five years, the roles are reversed—the crippling arthritis is now very controllable, and the good arthritis is difficult to treat due to government regulations!

***

That just about covers the FAQs. If you have a question that I didn't answer here, send me a message through my website at www.drsoloway.com. If you mention that you bought this book, I'll do my best to answer. In the meantime, check out my YouTube Channel. You'll probably find something useful there—and you'll definitely find something entertaining.

CHAPTER 15
PATIENT TESTIMONIALS

I've spent this entire book telling you why I'm the best. Still don't believe me? Check out what a few of my patients have to say, in their own words.

MARVEN CHIN

When I met Steve, around 1994, I was very sick. None of my doctors knew what was wrong with me. Basically, whenever I wasn't feeling well, they did lab work, and if they didn't know what it was, they'd tell me, "Marven, go admit yourself to the hospital." It was a lot easier to be admitted to the hospital back then.

Almost every weekend, I was going into the hospital because my doctors didn't know what to do. Sometimes they would do blood work and they would say, "Your blood work's fine," but I still felt horrible. They would question me, like, "Are you really sick?"

Other times, my blood work would be horrible, but I felt fine. They'd say, "Your blood work's bad, so you need to take this." Being young and naive, I would listen to the doctors, and whatever they prescribed, I would take—not knowing that some of the medication that they were giving me was actually making me much sicker.

I took it as prescribed, and I stopped it as prescribed. This actually created a lot more problems for my system. My body went into shock. In a one-year period, I was in the hospital at least two days, minimum, every month. It got to the point where I knew all the nurses.

One of the doctors would come in with shorts, flip-flops, a tank top, and a Hawaiian shirt and a stethoscope around his neck. He just didn't have the same professionalism. He would glance over some notes, look at me for like a minute if that, and say, "Okay, take this and then you're fine. Because, you know, I'm a doctor." If I ever questioned them, they would label me as nonconforming.

It just seemed like none of them knew what they were doing. I went from seeing a gastroenterologist, to an oncologist, and a surgical doctor—more than a dozen doctors, including other rheumatologists. They removed my spleen, and they removed my gallbladder. These were the prehistoric days when they would cut you up so you'd be out of commission for three weeks to two months. I didn't know what else they were going to cut out.

This was pre-Internet, so I started spending a lot of time in the library just trying to find an answer on my own. Over time, I began to realize that my problem was more rheumatological. I was working in Vineland, and I said, "You know what? I'm going to go see this doctor and share with him what I know, because every doctor that I've come across hasn't listened to me."

So far, the other doctors had treated me like a number. When I first went to see Steve, he treated me like a person. We talked for about an hour or so, and he diagnosed that I had an autoimmune disease. He was calm and reassuring. I said, "You know what? You're going to be my doctor." From then on to this day, almost twenty-six years, that's been true.

I've hardly ever had to go to the hospital again. My body still requires infusions, until the actual cure comes along. In the meantime, though, I've been able to have a normal life with work, a wife, and two kids thanks to Steve.

The first three or four years, we were just more like a doctor-patient relationship. Through the years, though, we started getting closer to the point where we'd go to basketball games with his son and my son, and all the way to the point when we went to China together and visited the Great Wall. We went to Hong Kong and Shanghai.

It's because of his influence that my son is now going to become a doctor. He's pretty much been following the career path that Steve laid out for him.

I can't say enough. I consider him to be like my brother, or even closer than some of my own family. He's just been there for me, and I know he's just a phone call away.

I love him like a brother, and he saved my life.

MARIA MASTROMATTEO

Steve and I went to high school together. He was on the swim team, and I was dating a guy who was on the swim team. He was so sweet, just like one of the nicest guys. Of course, he was always super smart, and very focused.

Years later, I was having some very bad health issues, and I reached out to him again. He couldn't have been better to me. It's a long story, but my doctors literally wanted me to have hand surgery. When I went to Steve, he just was like, "This is insane. You do not need hand surgery." He figured out the problem right away, and I didn't have to have surgery after all.

Steve started injecting my hands for me, and during one appointment his mother called probably ten times. Every time she'd call, he would answer, and talk to her very nicely, even though she obviously was interrupting. He's just so patient and has the perfect disposition to be a doctor.

I've never heard him raise his voice once, even though he's got a lot of patients and a lot going on in his office. He really cares about all his patients, and he really wants to help you—especially if no one else can figure it out. He will sit there and figure it out.

He actually did it twice for me, so I know firsthand that he doesn't just let things go. That's why when you go there, you may have to wait, but he's not in a rush. He wants to make sure that you're well taken care of. That's so rare in medicine these days. It's a business, like anything else now, but Steve has always been different. He just cares about his patients. It's not just because I know him; he's like this with everybody.

What a success story. His parents obviously did a great job with him, and they're very lucky to have somebody like that because, you know, a lot of people, they move on with their lives. They don't want to be bothered or whatever.

It's really quite something, what he's been able to achieve, and you know what? He's done it himself. His parents were good parents, but they weren't able to help him as much financially.

In high school, we were in a very affluent community. Everybody had like these big homes, and things like that. And he definitely didn't have that.

He wasn't one of the kids that had the, you know, BMW or anything. No. And I do remember he had to work, and most people in our high school did not have to do that.

He's completely self-made.

GEORGE KLINGOS

Back in 2007, I was with my wife in Greece, and she was diagnosed with ankylosing spondylitis. She was put on an injection every six weeks. We went to spend a few months in the States, and were looking for a rheumatologist to take care of her while we were there. We were recommended Dr. Soloway.

We thought that he'd just do the injections, but before, he said, "Just so I know what I'm doing, do you have anything from Greece? Any kind of blood work, so I'll know you actually do have ankylosing spondylitis?" We get the blood work and scan, and he says, "This is all clear. It doesn't show any of that."

My wife was shocked. Dr. Soloway said that what they'd told her had been all wrong, misdiagnoses. He said, "I don't know what your wife has, but I know what she does not have that is spondylitis." As we went on, he diagnosed that she most likely had drug-induced lupus, so he treated her for that and made her well. The bigger problem, though, was most likely something called fibromyalgia. Dr. Soloway saved her life. She would be dead if she stayed in Greece or went to another doctor here in the States.

Because of our experience, we became friends, and I invited him to come to Greece as a thank-you for what he had done for my wife. Within one week, he saw more than most people can see in a month. In addition, he saw so many local patients that needed medical care—even though it was his vacation!

While we were going around sightseeing, people were calling me and asking me, "Do you mind asking your friend?" about this and that. We came back from Athens at one o'clock in the morning, and people came in to see him. One of them was suffering from psoriatic arthritis. So, he brought the blood work. He brought, you know, the medication he was taking. Steve takes one look at the medication and tells me he should not be taking it because it's going to make his blood pressure go crazy. I was the translator as he taught him to get on Remicade. Steve said to wait until the summer and the majority of his problems would go away. That's exactly the way it happened.

The next day, we were supposed to leave for the airport. There was enough time left to take a walk around the city, but we could not do that because for three hours, people were coming to the house to be seen by Steve. He was not rude or dismissive to anyone. He was patiently explaining to everyone about their condition and what to do. He's just always helping people. People still remember what he did for them. It's just unbelievable.

All of my friends in the States whom I've referred to him have come back and thanked me. They say, "We've never seen somebody that could treat the condition we had so well." I remember a friend came to me—a six-foot-two, fifty-year-old guy—in tears with pain. He could not sleep all night because of pain in his hand, his shoulder.

After he had a couple of shots, Dr. Soloway told him, "Twist your arm, and twist your shoulder. You know, start moving it." The guy almost wanted to hit Steve! He was like, "You're bullshitting me if you're telling me to move it." He gives it a shot, starts moving slowly, and before he knew it, he could swing his arm around like nothing. He couldn't believe it.

Steve is a miracle worker.

CARLEEN DIPAOLA

About fifteen years ago, I was a patient of Dr. Soloway's. Like so many other patients, I absolutely fell in love with the doctor because he made me feel better. He totally cured me.

For three years, I had lived in terrible pain from neck issues, and my quality of life just wasn't there. He gave me back my quality of life, and for that I will be forever grateful.

He can be so understanding and sympathetic, whereas you wouldn't necessarily think that when you first meet him. When you first meet him, you're just like, "This guy isn't sympathetic at all! This guy just says it the way it is." Whether you like it or not, it's actually a great thing that he is so honest and direct. Plus, he does have that inner level of sweetness and empathy and kindness—but he doesn't share that with everybody.

At the time that Dr. Soloway was treating me, I was involved in local politics here in Cumberland County. Dr. Soloway frequently was invited to political events and things of that nature, so we continued to cross paths and keep in touch.

A new administration had come in, and I lost my job. While I was browsing the ads, I saw that Dr. Soloway was offering a position as a personal assistant. The business administrator, Debra, interviewed me and told me what my duties would be, and I accepted the position. Dr. Soloway told me what he expected from me, and here I am a year later.

As his personal administrative assistant, I do whatever the doctor needs, the way it needs to be done. Not only do I take care of personal things for Dr. Soloway, such as his travel, keeping track of his medical board meetings, scheduling all of his meetings; but also, I do anything that his parents need done, like ordering things. I help his children at times, as well. I research medical items that he may want to order. Really, I do anything that Dr. Soloway wants me to do.

As a patient of his, I had grown a lot of respect for Dr. Soloway and for what he has done. Working alongside him in the political realm, working with him now, the only thing I can say is that the man is absolutely brilliant. I'm just a fan. The transition from patient to personal assistant was a little bit of a transition, but in the end it was easy.

He's so great to work for. He treats all of us fair, but he expects the work to be done correctly, of course. He's a stickler for that, obviously, because it's his practice. He's very matter-of-fact. He knows what he wants and he wants what he wants and he will get what he wants. That's it. So, whatever he wants is fine with me, and I try my best to do it.

Luckily, the more I work, the more I seem to know exactly what he wants. I'm almost to the point where I know he wants something before he even tells me. It feels really good to anticipate his needs. I can say, "It's already done!" and get no response. So then, I know that's good. It's just about being in tune with him, to the environment, to the type of day he had, especially if he was swamped.

Perhaps the greatest reason why I love my job is because he treats the people around him like family, whether it's patients or employees. When it comes to his real family, he is a very big family man. He visits his parents daily, no matter how tired he is and how long he's worked. Even if it's been a ten- or eleven-hour day, he'll still go over to see his mom and dad, who really enjoy those visits.

As his staff, we kind of treat him like family, too. He loves celebrating his birthday. Of course, we always know it's coming, but he doesn't know *how* it's coming in any given year. We usually decorate the break room for him and everybody gets together toward the end of the day when the patients are gone, and we have a cake. This year, we decided to do something a little different, and we decorated his office.

It all worked out perfectly. Dr. Soloway had to go up to Trenton for a Board of Medical Examiners meeting, and we got to work. We had banners, streamers, and balloons hanging from the walls and the ceiling. There was a huge "Happy Birthday" sign, and two big mylar balloons showing his age.

We had somebody hiding in his bathroom so we could get his initial reaction when he first opened up the door, and he was so surprised and happy. He kept it up for the whole month of February! We weren't allowed to take it down. I said, "Doc, you want me to take care of this?" and he said, "No. Don't touch it until I ask you to."

By the end of two weeks, all the balloons were on the ground and just the banner was still up, so he finally let us take it all down. It was great to be able to do something like that, because he is so thoughtful and caring; he'll do anything for anyone.

Somehow, he manages to balance that with the fact that he's running a business and it's not a playground. It's a very lucrative business, at that.

I just love everything that he has taught me. Knowing him has made me better.

RV TURNER

About thirty years ago, I broke my back. I was supposed to never walk again, but I got steel rods in my back and went back to work. I was a roofer, and I went back to roofing even though the doctors told me not to. Before long, my knees were shot along with my back, and I was taking somewhere around ninety-five Percocets a month. It wasn't an addiction, because some days I'd take none, and some days I'd take ten. I was a roofer, and I needed to work. If I didn't work, the bills didn't get paid. What was I supposed to do? Go live off of twelve hundred dollars a month in disability?

At one point, I was working for a guy who saw how much pain I was in, and told me, "Go see Dr. Soloway." So, I made an appointment and got there at ten o'clock in the morning. By the time I saw him, it was 3:30 p.m. He was really my last chance.

Doc couldn't believe the work that I did, that I was doing it the way my back was. He started off by giving me four shots in my back, a facet joint injection. I felt better that day, and I haven't had to take any pain medication since—except Aleve on rainy days. I also get a shot maybe once a year in each knee.

Not everyone in my position actually wants to get better, I've learned. Doc told me, "I get people who come in here and all they say is that they want me to sign off so they can get disability. They don't want to work."

It's so true. When I was in what they call pain management, I used to hear from people all the time, "Don't go to Dr. Soloway. He won't give you pain pills."

"Don't go to Dr. Soloway. He won't give you disability."

Doc wants you to get better. He wants to cure you, so you don't need these things. Those people were bums just looking around to get disability or get pills.

That's how the system is broken, right? They all sat in that office and they were telling each other what doctor to go see: "He'll give you disability. He'll give you pain medication. Don't go to Dr. Soloway, because he won't give you either."

If you actually want to get better, Doc is the one to see. I've seen him treat people without any insurance, who can't pay, just to help them get better. He's not in it for the money. He enjoys his work and he wants to make people better.

I've recommended all my uncles, my father, friends, and so many people. I tell them, "You might wait a little while, but when you leave, you will be feeling better. He's really life-changing."

When I met Doc, I was ready to give up, but he gave me my life back. Everybody I know has gotten knee replacements, and my doctors were urging me to do that too, to go on permanent disability. Instead, I'm still working. I cut trees; I do painting; I do siding. I'm doing all of that for Dr. Soloway, too.

At my appointment, when he asked me what I did, I said, "roofing and general contracting."

He took my number down and said, "I'm gonna have my lady call you," because they were looking for some help. To start, he got me to work one day a week. Then, it was two days a week, three days a week, and so on. I've worked seven days a week for doc for the last seven or eight years.

I've been all over the country with Doc, and working for him. He took me to the White House to meet President Trump. I met Lou Ferrigno, baseball all-stars, and more. He took me to New York, for a $26 hamburger! He gave me the keys to his Bentley, a $300,000 car, to go pick it up for him and drive it home, all by myself. I have keys to all of his properties.

I consider him my best friend, and there isn't anything I wouldn't do for him. If he called me at two, three o'clock in the morning and said, "I need your help," I'd be there in a minute. He saved my life.

CHRISTOPHER LOTZ

I drive all the way from Louisiana up to New Jersey to get my injections from Dr. Soloway. I don't especially like to do it, but he's the only one who's ever been able to give me relief. I tried to find a doctor down here who would just give me the same treatment as he does, but they blew me off because he is a Caribbean med school grad.

With COVID-19, I haven't been able to get up there, because I've made the choice to avoid immunosuppression.

It's hard, but it just makes me realize how grateful I am to Dr. Soloway. It's too bad our government was asleep at the wheel and let this happen.

TOM BRADY

Steve and I met at a gym. We both worked out in the mornings, and we became friends after running into each other and talking and so forth. I started to use him as a resource whenever I needed some medical information, or referrals, or just a little guidance. To say the least, it was the best thing that ever happened to me.

I have so many examples that explain why. In just one incident, I had to go for a chest X-ray for something; I don't remember what. The physician that did the X-ray—a physician who was *not* affiliated with Steve—either inadvertently read it wrong or mixed up whatever the case was and told me I had terminal lung cancer.

I was stunned. My first resource to go to was Steve. Of course, he immediately laid out the protocol for me: This is where you need to go, what you have to do. He got me in to see a specialist early.

Nine days later, I was at the Fox Chase Cancer Center outside Philadelphia. I went through the whole litany of testing only to find out that, no, I had nothing. The local physician was just totally inept. I mean, anybody can make a mistake, but he didn't return my call for three days after I let him know that what he told me wasn't true. Then, he had his secretary call me and say that I could come to his office and he would apologize to me. It was just beyond belief.

I mean, I was walking around my house, telling my wife, "This is how you turn off the sprinkler system. This is what you have to do in winter." I mean, these are all the things you go through when you think that everything around the corner is going to happen to you.

In another example, I got a call from my son saying that he had gone to the hospital because he had jaundice, and the testing came back saying he had a mass on the pancreas. Right away, I thought it was pancreatic cancer.

So again, I went to Steve and explained the situation. Steve not only laid out everything that we had to do, but also, he made phone calls at like eleven, twelve o'clock at night to physicians he thought that my son should see.

Six days after my son was diagnosed, he was in surgery. It turned out it was not cancerous, but he still had a Whipple surgery, which is a massively invasive surgery. They basically go in and just gut you all around. He's recovered today. Without Steve's guidance, I would have been lost.

Steve relishes the challenge of medicine. Right away, he'll take it on: how do I solve the problem? Whatever it takes, he thinks outside the box to solve it. He's like Dr. House without the attitude problems. In fact, somebody way back gave him all of the seasons of *House* to watch, because he didn't know who House was at the time and they said, this is who you are.

Beyond that, I just really enjoy his company. His intellect is bar none, just terrific. When we go out to dinner, the conversation is always enlightening. It's refreshing. I can't say enough about the guy.

For Steve, I'd do anything. I mean, literally anything. I told him that. I mean, for what he's done for me and my family? Without a doubt, I'd do anything. We're lucky to have him.

CAROL

Steve and I knew each other from the gym. My husband's into martial arts, so he was always getting beat up and had back problems. Steve shot him up, and they developed a great relationship. Then we started training Steve in the martial arts, too, and he eventually got a black belt.

We became really great friends. When Steve's son turned eight or nine, he had a party for his family, and my husband cut a lettuce on Steve's stomach with a machete.

He's a great guy. I broke my leg, and we didn't have medical insurance at the time. He took some X-rays, and he goes, "Yeah, it's broken."

I was like, "Oh, I'm a black belt. I'll tough it out."

But he's like, "No, you got to see an orthopedic surgeon."

I said, "Well, I don't have medical insurance, so that's not going to happen." He gave me an air cast and crutches, and I was on my way.

Another time, my husband had cancer, and Steve would call up just to make sure everything was fine and see if he needed anything.

Steve goes 100 percent no matter what it is he does. He loves being a doctor. He loves patients. He loves to see people get healed. When he does martial arts, you can't tell him to tone it down because he doesn't know how. It's 100 percent or nothing. And that goes for everything he does. It's like, if you're not going to do it 100 percent, then don't do it. He doesn't slack on anything.

We'll be friends for life.

CANDACE SHELSON, BSN, RN

(The following is an actual office note—included here before Shelson's testimonial).

> Shelson, Candace—Date of service 10-04-2016
>
> I reviewed the documented medical, surgical, family, social, medication, drug allergy and immunization histories.
>
> **Plan**
>
> While I cannot prove her diagnosis without a biopsy, it is very suspicious for malignancy and without further ado this patient must have a bone marrow biopsy; and if the bone marrow biopsy fails to show a malignancy, I would then recommend a skin biopsy of normal skin to look for intravascular lymphoma. It would be very easy to start this patient on Rituximab anticipating a great response to therapy, but with no diagnosis I would be doing the patient a very grave disservice in the future. At this time, I feel that the patient is being dealt a raw deal and being pushed off. She actually asked for a bone marrow biopsy and then was told that it

could not be done because the facility she goes to had run out of bone marrow kits. I made suggestions to the patient other than AtlantiCare, where she should go to have a bone marrow biopsy and then be treated properly. Once again, her cryoglobulins were ordered. My fear is that she could have type I cryoglobulins that would be associated with her C-reactive protein of 24, which is significantly elevated, monoclonal protein 0.5 with IgG monoclonal protein and light chains, and Bence Jones protein in the urine sample. I am not aware of any disease other than a malignancy that would cause this picture and I do believe her underlying disease presented in a vasculitic manner with digital infarctions that h e a le d on steroids and migratory polyarthritis. She fortunately did change primary care physicians as she was very disgruntled with the first who was bold enough to tell her not to come here. Also noted is her mild atherosclerotic disease at the origin of the left subclavian artery, which in fact does not explain any of her features as she had infarcts in both hands. In addition, her thyroid nodules have been biopsied and have been benign. Contrary to the oncologist telling the patient that there is no malignancy, I strongly disagree with this and I do not think that an assessment of whether she has one or not can be made for sure without this biopsy; and if she has to leave the AtlantiCare system that she is mandated to go to, I believe and would encourage her to get legal counsel because of the care she has had up until this point does not meet the standard care. Flu vaccine administered without complication. Greater than 75 minutes face-to-face time was spent with the patient. This is a summary of the discussion with the patient and in no way is intended to be a verbatim summation of everything discussed.

It all started back in June of 2016, when I started becoming very ill. I had a fine needle biopsy, and my thyroid began experiencing symptoms after that.

It apparently caused a pretty bad infection. I was healthy prior to that, a sixty-one-year-old healthy individual.

I had researched it at the time even to find out what was going on with me, and it's one of those very rare side effects that you would get from having a biopsy done this way. By the end of June, I wasn't feeling right. My hands were turning red, white, and black. Of course, everybody wanted to attribute that to Raynaud's disease. I left work and went to my primary care because my left knee had swollen up and I could hardly even walk. The primary care did some blood work. Of course, they all came back normal. She didn't care that I couldn't ambulate. She didn't even look. She had some medical assistant who wasn't even a nurse look at me. I don't know what their background was.

Two days after I had seen her, I had to go to urgent care because nothing was getting better and I was in pain. I could take pain, but it was like nothing I had ever experienced. She did a Lyme disease test and of course gave me a prescription for Naproxen, and we went along from there.

Soon, I started losing weight. I wasn't feeling good. I was still fatigued. I just know my body, and I knew something was wrong.

One of the girls I work with said, "You know, I go to this doctor who's great. Nobody's helping you. You need to go see him."

So, in two weeks I had an appointment with him. Before I left, he told me that I had a life-threatening illness and that he was going to find out what it was. In the meantime, while he was seeing me that night, he took blood out of my left knee. He injected my left arm, which I couldn't even move. He put me on prednisone and gave me orders for tests to be done.

A lot of the tests, the first series of tests that he ran, came back negative. He decided to do more. Those tests came back negative. He decided to do more. In the meantime, there were other things going on. Like I had to take some lab tests to urgent care. They screwed those up completely.

At the end of July, Soloway says, "I'm urging you to go seek help. I think you have melanoma."

I call the cancer institute that's associated with where I work and my insurance. I finally get an appointment with them. I walked in, they have the lab results Dr. Soloway ran, and the woman says to me upon meeting me and just looking at the lab results, "I don't know why he would tell you that you have cancer. You don't have cancer."

She hasn't done an assessment. She hasn't done a thing. He was so upset, he actually wrote me a letter to sue them.

I was just like, "Okay. I'm thrilled to death. I don't have cancer."

But Dr. Soloway said, "I'm telling you to get a bone marrow biopsy right now. You need to go back and tell them you need to go tomorrow to get a biopsy."

I called them, we set it up, and they called me back two weeks later. They said, "We ran out of bone marrow biopsy kits." This is a cancer center.

I'm like, "I don't have cancer," so it moves on, even though my hands are still turning red.

They did follow up with one of the cardiologists, and he said, "You know, I know you're sixty and you have no high blood pressure, no cholesterol. You're very, very low risk for cardiovascular disease."

That being said, I called the cancer center back, and I finally scheduled the bone marrow biopsy with this doctor. They do it. She calls me back a couple of weeks later and says, "You have Non-Hodgkin's Lymphoma."

Dr. Soloway diagnosed me in July. They didn't diagnose me until November. He could not believe that all this time went by.

He is phenomenal because he doesn't give up. Everyone else blew me off because my presentation was good. As a nurse, I knew I was really sick. I knew something was wrong, and he figured it out. He's phenomenal.

The people whom I've sent to him feel the same way. Somebody else I worked with, her husband had been diagnosed with gout forever. He went to Dr. Soloway, and he found out it wasn't gout.

I don't know what's going on in the medical field, but people just, for lack of a better term, they blow you off. I really didn't have a relationship with any physician, and Dr. Soloway just took me under his wing. I could see him actually thinking about my answers and where he was going to go next with his questions. I was smart enough to keep my mouth shut and just answer his questions and let him do what he does best. He said, "You have a life-threatening emergency and I am going to find out what it is because nobody else is helping you." And he did.

To top it all off, my insurance wouldn't pay for it, so he wrote that off and has not charged me a thing. What doctor does that? He's phenomenal.

TROY BURGER

I gotta give you the whole story if you want the whole story. I live in South Jersey, and I own a repair shop. It's a tough business, and you get aggravated with your employees.

Everything was good until sometime in my forties, I woke up one night and I could actually feel my heartbeat in my temples. At the time, my wife was working in the ER. She was really medically savvy as far as the fact that she was in the ER trauma center all the time. Me, I don't go to doctors. I don't go to the hospital. Like, you gotta cut my hand off before I go anywhere. That night, she heard me get up and she's like, "What's the matter?"

I said, "I don't feel right." I went to take a shower and it didn't go away. She went into panic mode. So, I ended up in the ER even though I didn't have any chest pain or anything. I just had this rapid-fire heartbeat and I could hear it in my ears, and I could see my temples going crazy.

By the time I got to see someone, it had stopped. But the girl who triaged me took my blood pressure anyway, and she was like, "Do you feel all right?"

I'm like, "Yeah."

She says, "You don't have any pain?"

And I'm like, "No." The next thing I know, she grabs this mic, and she's like, "Cardiology stat, cardiology stat."

I'm like, "What the hell is going on?"

My wife looks at me and goes, "Your blood pressure's two-oh-one." Like okay, well is that bad or good? Apparently, that's bad. Like, you're going to stroke or have a heart attack bad. I was in there from two in the morning until ten in the morning, just want to get my blood pressure down.

After that, they told me to go to the cardiologist. I go in there, and my blood pressure was high. The doctor says, "What can we do to get the blood pressure down?"

And I'm like, "Really? You're the cardiologist. I'll tell you what you can do. Write me a check for $250,000. I guarantee you my blood pressure will go down." You know what I mean? I was aggravated. Why was he asking *me* what to do?

He gave me some meds, and not long after that I started having anxiety attacks. I couldn't sleep at night. I had to be in bed sitting up because I had such bad acid reflux. I told my wife, "Go make sure the life insurance is ready. My ass is dying."

I went back to the cardiologist. He did an EKG stress test, and he put me on twelve pills a day. Here I go from not even taking an aspirin when I have a headache, and this guy has got me on twelve pills a day.

So, I went back to him and I said, "Listen, I'm getting terrible heartburn and these anxiety attacks."

He started telling me, "Well, you gotta lose some weight. You know, I think a lot of it's in your head. I think you're making it out worse than what it is. Your heart looks really good."

He kept doing all this testing and said, "Well, you're actually doing great. Your blood pressure's coming down a little bit."

I'm like, "This is good? I'm strong, and I don't even want to get out of my chair because I'm so exhausted from having panic attacks and this acid reflux." I didn't know what to do.

At the time, my brother-in-law was a builder, with like forty guys under him. He had to go to the hospital, and the hospital didn't follow protocol, so he ended up with some kind of brain seizures. My sister was taking him to every doctor along the East Coast trying to get him straightened out, because they had a million-dollar business about to go down the drain, because he couldn't work. I told them what was going on, and she said I should go see Dr. Soloway. She said, you know, "Prepare yourself, because this guy is gonna blast you. He doesn't play games. He's going to fight you."

And I'm like, "Whatever, I gotta do something. I don't know what else to do. But why are you having me go to an arthritis doctor?"

She said, "Troy, there was nothing he could do for Ed, but I'm going to tell you right now. I've been to every doctor on the East Coast. This guy is like Dr. House."

She said, "He looked at me and was like, 'You have a goiter in your neck.' I was like, this guy's a quack."

"He didn't even feel my neck or look at me or anything," she said, but a few weeks later she ended up in the hospital, and whatever he said she had, she had. It was crazy.

Finally, I get in to see him. He comes in, says hi, and from that moment on, we became really good friends. He's a straight shooter, and I want somebody to be straight to me, you know?

The cardiologist wasn't. He'd said that out of all the medicine he was giving me, none of it would cause acid reflux. Well, when I went to pick up my prescriptions one day, I asked the pharmacist, "Do any of these cause acid reflux?"

The pharmacist is like, "Well, this one causes acid reflux, and this one." Why would the doctor tell me that none of the medicines caused acid reflux? That pissed me off. You know what I'm saying? That really pissed me off.

When I got to Dr. Soloway, I got in there and he talked to me probably for about half hour to an hour. He asked me what I did for living, dah, dah, dah. He was prying. I had my wife with me, and she kept looking at me because she knew he was kind of prying, but he was just trying to find out what the situation was, you know what I'm saying?

He showed me the lab for blood work and takes about a gallon of blood from me. The lab girl said, "I want to tell you right now, he's checking you for everything from AIDS to Lyme disease."

I was supposed to go back to him two or three days later, and before the appointment he had a girl call from the office and tell me to bring all of my prescriptions.

They checked my blood and they checked my weight again. He comes in, he looks at my chart, and he sits down. He says, "Well, I think I might know what the problem is."

And I said, "Really?!"

He said, "Yeah. Your number one problem is that your cardiologist is an asshole." This is the truth.

He said, "Where are your prescriptions?" My wife had them all set on the counter and I swear to you, he grabbed the trash can and pushed everything in the trash can.

He said, "You're going to go to the pharmacy and you're going to buy a one milligram Bayer aspirin. I'm going to put you on Nexium, and you're going to take a time-release dose of Xanax."

I was like, "Dude, I'm not taking that."

He said, "Listen, don't be asinine. It's not a Percocet. It's not Oxycontin. It's just going to level you out. You are going through what every other business owner's going through. There's nothing wrong with your heart."

He said, "Your blood pressure issue is not caused by heart problems. Your blood pressure was caused by other organs in your body. Furthermore, you're going to get tested for sleep apnea because you've got sleep apnea."

I said, "Well, how do you know that?"

He said, "Because I can look at you and see you've got sleep apnea."

The next thing I know, after about three weeks, my blood pressure is 121 over 70 and I'm happy."

We became friends, and after a few years, he said, "I'm not trying to scare you, but you're getting to be about that age that you should probably see a cardiologist."

So I go back, and he pulls me off everything Dr. Soloway had me on and gives me other pills. Here comes the acid reflux back again. My blood pressure went up again. My anxiety's off the walls. Every time I go see him, the guy's telling me I'm doing great, but I have to see him every three weeks, so I can't be doing too great. When Dr. Soloway found out, he called the guy and flipped out. I trust him.

Then, I started getting stomach pains. I don't know what to do, and I don't want to bother Dr. Soloway with it because he's a rheumatologist, but like I said, I trust him.

I go back to Dr. Soloway, and he says, "I'm going to send you for an ultrasound. I think you have a gallbladder problem."

Well, he sent me for an ultrasound, and the day he sent me to the ultrasound, he went to Israel. In the meantime, my gallbladder erupted and sepsis went through my whole body.

I ended up in the ER, and the last thing I remember was drinking a glass of Tang and I don't remember another thing after that. I was in intensive care for eleven days. The doctors told my wife, "Listen, you might want to make arrangements. We don't know if he's going to come through this." My liver shut down, my pancreas shut down, and she didn't know what to do.

My general practitioner was useless. So, she called Dr. Soloway. Dr. Soloway called in from Israel, and even though he was on vacation, he called my wife every single day. My wife was going to pull me out of there, and he told her to wait until he could talk to my doctors.

He called my doctors, called my wife back, said, "Leave him right there. He's got one of the best surgeons working on him. Just stay right there. He's going to be fine. I'll be home in three more days." He was, and I pulled through.

Listen, his nickname is MacGyver. He'll do anything to get to the bottom of what's bothering you. He's an Einstein, a mad scientist. The bottom line is, if he can't figure it out in twenty-four hours, he'll find you someone who can.

A LOCAL INSURANCE CONSULTANT

He's a genius, actually. I mean, he is crazy, but he can diagnose things by you just telling him the symptoms. Or even if he looks at you, which is incredible. I'm not kidding.

My wife was feeling really horrible. She's a little thing. She's only five foot, two and 110 pounds. And she started bloating in her abdominal area. We admitted her into the hospital. And my friend that's a cardiologist was treating her in the hospital and there were, you know, ten other doctors, literally.

For almost a week, they could not figure out what was going on with her. She kept swelling, and fluid was filling the space around the heart (pericardial space). We started getting really nervous. She was feeling horrible. She was bloated and she is a perfectly healthy person. I happen to see Steve at the gym. And I said, "Doc, this is driving me crazy."

He said, "Tell me her symptoms." I said, "She's bloated," that kind of thing.

He said, "You know, let me ask you something. If you walked by a building and it was on fire, what would you do?"

I said, "I'd get water and put it out!"

He said, "So has anybody brought in an inflammatory disease doctor? She needs to get the inflammation out before anything is going to be right."

He couldn't give her steroids since he wasn't her doctor, but he said, "Go back and tell them that. Just recommend that she maybe try steroids because nothing else was working." I go back to the doctor, and the doctor got all twisted and said no to the steroids.

Finally, a week's time went by and I said to my wife, "We're getting you out of here."

She was stable, but she was still bloated. I got her home and Dr. Soloway prescribed what she had to have and in a matter of probably thirty-six hours, she was back to normal.

These are the kind of things that he does. He's just a genius.

At the same time, this is my thirty-ninth year as an insurance consultant, which encompasses health insurance, dental, prescription vision. We have a lot in common with Doc Soloway, because our job for our clients is to get them the right benefits in the most cost-effective way we can.

From the standpoint of being a health insurance provider, the problem with a lot of things going on nowadays is everybody's kind of thinking of health insurance and treatment as if they're going to McDonald's for fast food. People say, "Well, I could get this surgery and in six months I'll be back to normal." Well, no. That's a seventy-, eighty-thousand-dollar surgery. They'd rather take that "easy" route rather than say, "Well, you know what? If my back's sore, I'll go work out and get my abdominal area stronger to help it."

Dr. Soloway is a firm believer in trying to avoid surgeries and unnecessary treatments. It's not the norm for the industry, but I am a firm believer in what he does.

A VERY SUCCESSFUL INTERNATIONAL BUSINESSMAN WHO KNOWS ME WELL

I first met Dr. Soloway when we were neighbors in the same Miami Beach apartment building. Although we have different backgrounds, we share similar interests and views.

Aside from his medical prowess, he is a very smart and shrewd businessman. His keen sense of timing with regard to investments exemplifies his business expertise. I am impressed that someone so committed to his medical practice can also be a successful investor.

He adheres to a strict daily regimen that allows him time for his patients first and foremost but also provides him time to swim daily for his own physical health. Even during a personal health crisis, his physical and mental health were priorities. He can definitely use more vacation time!

His family and his patients are of utmost importance to him. I look up to Dr. Soloway; even though we are not close in age, we have a mutual respect and a lot to learn from each other.

***

These are just a few of the thousands of raving reviews that I have received over the years. My Yelp page and Facebook page are full of them. I can't even post on Facebook without someone adding a new one in the comments! If you ever find yourself in need of rheumatological treatment, reach out. I would love to have your story in my next book!

CHAPTER 16
THE MEANING OF SUCCESS

I've come a long way from Corona, Queens. Instead of riding a bike through a slum, I live in a home, close to my parents and children. I drive the car to work, no more hitchhiking, and this gives me, in one aspect, a feeling of achievement.

As a result of hard work, and through my practice, I've been able to feed many families of hard workers. *Without my **dedicated**, hardworking staff, I would never have achieved the success that would have been unknown to me in my earlier life.*

The field of medicine has provided me with a very fulfilling career. I have been blessed. At forty years old, I was the youngest person to be named to Castle Connolly's Top Docs list, published in *Philadelphia* magazine. I've been a perennial addition to the list ever since—and that's not because I am the most handsome and have the coolest shirts. I haven't been able to snag the cover. When I inquired, I was notified that physicians *aren't normally shown* on the cover. This is a blatant lie, as many docs have adorned the cover.

In writing this book, I went back to my old mentor and dear friend, Dr. Larry Leventhal, and asked him if my life has lived up to the dreams, goals, and vision I had shared with him in the early days of my rise to the top. This is what he had to say:

I always view my students as almost like my kids, you know? I'm happy for their success, because I feel I played a role in IT. Steve has earned everything that he has obtained—as far as financially, politically, whatever—through hard work.

Unfortunately, the more you're in the public eye and the more successful you become, you're sometimes a target of people who want to say, "Well, you know, he's more successful than me because he got this break or he did something he shouldn't have done." That kind of thing. That's happened to Steve. (That said, twenty-five years ago, I was harassed by one of his local haters, long before his huge successes. Remember I covered his practice for two separate weeks and quit due to exhaustion.)

I have always supported him and said, "Look, as long as you're not doing anything immoral or illegal, then you just work hard and become successful." I didn't even have to tell him because he was always that kind of individual. He's a very bright guy, with very high energy.

Success can be defined in many different ways. If you're happy as an individual, you're successful. It doesn't matter how much money you make or how many accolades you get or awards you win. Your success should be self-determined. For Steve, success was never failing at anything he did. And as his mentor, I can assure you nobody worked harder or asked more questions. He put in what it took to be the superb physician that he grew into. (He's a great guy, too.) He is the best fellow I trained!

I always expected him to be successful, but he's certainly gone beyond that. (He is the face of Rheumatology in New Jersey.) You can't predict if somebody is going to go to an area that's underserved and revolutionize the rheumatology field in an area that never had a rheumatologist. Steve could've just gone there and opened up a little private practice and seen the normal number of patients, but he took it to another level.

I met his mother once at one of his kid's birthday parties and his parents are very down-to-earth, unassuming individuals. I remember talking to his mom at this party, and she said, "I don't know where he gets his drive. He's so much more motivated than we were and has so much more desire to be successful than we cared about."

Today, we are both busy in our independent lives, but we are close friends, he is like a great brother to me. He *loves* discussing interesting cases (lifetime student of the field) that he finds interesting or he'll call me up for help with a case. I do the same to him. That's what good doctors do. We don't know everything, and we want to have a second pair of ears and eyes on a case. What do you think? What should I do? This kind of thing. That's the ongoing greatness that you want every doctor to have. You want every doctor to never stop asking questions. Steve's always been the younger brother I never had.

Even the best, I continue asking myself how I can continue improving each day—from my patient care, to hitting a new personal best with my swimming or Peloton.

Sharing my knowledge is a wonderful feeling. I have mentored many peers and students over the years. This book is an extension of that. I trust you've gained helpful insights, regardless of where you are in your life. I hope this book empowers you as you may have to deal with the system—unknowingly, or at any time. Even better, stay healthy and avoid me at all cost!

ACKNOWLEDGMENTS

Without the unwavering and unconditional love bestowed upon me by my amazing parents, Frances and Warren, there would be no book. "Go where your life will be the best, we will follow you there."

My children, Alyxandra and Jacob, with pride I instill strong values and teach you the virtue of why daddy comes home late too often.

Without these men, I would not have the tools to be in my own shoes: M. Anthony Albornoz, MD (piqued my interest); Bruce Hoffman, MD (made it real); H. R. Schumacher, Jr., MD (most inquisitive); Lawrence Leventhal, MD (kept it fun).

To my best friends and coworkers, your timeless devotion can't be measured: David Weksel; Robert Feferman, MD; Kurt Henry, MD (DK Star Productions); Debra Richards, CEO; Denise Lister, CMA; Dana Solomon, CMA; Audrey Rubano, NP (proof I am a Rheum fellowship); Julia Tillman; and Tim Lieske.

And finally, Martin Koslin (love you Uncle Martin).